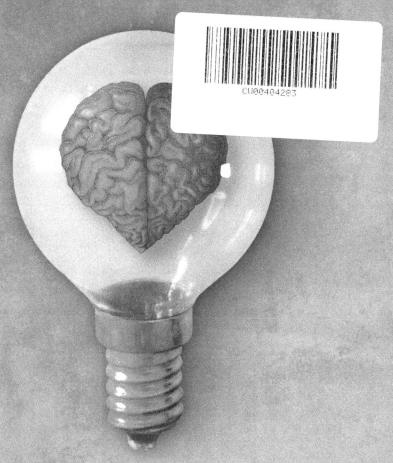

USE YOUR HEAD
HEAL YOUR HEART

HOW TO AVOID OR RECOVER
FROM HEART DISEASE!

SEAN FANE

ISBN 978-1-8384783-0-8 (Paperback)

ISBN 978-1-8384783-1-5 (ebook)

ISBN 978-1-8384783-2-2 (PDF)

Written, indexed and designed by Sean Fane

Cover design by Christopher Gibbs

Cartoons by YSFWORKS

With special thanks to Ed Cordin and Julie Wilson for editing guidance, and encouragement.

For my loves, Elliot, Phoebe and Dubs

CONTENTS

INTRODUCTION

"If you were to line-up 100 people of your age in a room, you are pretty much the last person I would have expected to have a heart attack!"

More than 17 million people per year die from cardiovascular disease [1] (CVD) globally, and two years ago I was very nearly one of them, yet I was not considered high-risk by my doctor.

The encouraging words at the top of the page were from my cardiologist on the first check-up after my heart attack.

He didn't know why I had atherosclerosis, and surprisingly to me, he didn't plan to investigate the cause.

As we approach middle age it is increasingly likely that we will know somebody that has been affected by heart disease.

It seems to me that we see heart disease as almost an inevitability, part of the ageing process, and something that we should be conscious of "trying", but ultimately failing, to avoid throughout our lives.

And this isn't surprising, as coronary heart disease (CHD) is the leading cause of death in the Western world.

However, until a little over a century ago, heart disease was almost unheard of.

---

[1]   https://academic.oup.com/eurheartj/article/37/42/3232/2536403

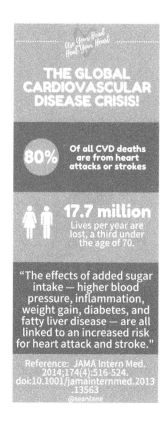

THE GLOBAL CARDIOVASCULAR DISEASE CRISIS!

80% Of all CVD deaths are from heart attacks or strokes

17.7 million Lives per year are lost, a third under the age of 70.

"The effects of added sugar intake — higher blood pressure, inflammation, weight gain, diabetes, and fatty liver disease — are all linked to an increased risk for heart attack and stroke."

Reference: JAMA Intern Med. 2014;174(4):516-524. doi:10.1001/jamainternmed.2013 .13563
@seanfane

Before gyms were operating in every town, before middle-aged men filled the roads in lycra-clad peletons, before we started counting calories, before we panicked about LDL levels (before we even knew what LDL was), before we had "fat-free" versions of popular foods, before skimmed milk, before we legislated for food packaging information, before we had blood-pressure medication, before statins….before all of these things……heart disease was negligible.

Practically non-existent.

Furthermore, incidences of diabetes were extremely rare, and cancer incidence was significantly lower too.

Modern chronic diseases, as they have come to be collectively termed, are just that. Modern. They haven't been around for very long.

So how, after 200,000 years of existing on earth, have humans gone from a species that dies from old-age, bacterial infections, viruses, accidents and child-birth for 199,880-ish years, to one that mainly dies from heart disease, diabetes and cancer in the last 120 years?

Despite the advancements in hygiene, science and medicine that have enabled us to combat or eradicate some of our most feared bacterial and infectious diseases, these modern chronic diseases are becoming more and more prevalent.

Surely our advances in technology and medicine have some clues for us, to help us to understand what we are doing so badly wrong?

We have never known more about food and nutrition.

We have never known more about exercise and wellness.

We have never known more about chemistry, physics and biology.

We have never had such amazing technology to enable us to improve health outcomes.

And despite all of this, we have allowed ourselves to become fatally afflicted by chronic disease.

Not only that, but the dietary, lifestyle and medication advice that we adopt certainly isn't working.

How is this possible, and what can you do to prevent yourself from adding to the statistics, by 'sleep-walking' into cardiovascular disease?

HOW I CAME TO WRITE THIS BOOK

After experiencing a near fatal heart attack at 51, with low cholesterol and with no obvious risk-factors, I was fitted with a stent and prescribed a life-sentence of medication, most of which held the promise of some pretty awful side effects.

I was surprised to discover that the cardiology team at the hospital that treated me didn't know why I had suffered a heart attack, and didn't intend to investigate the cause either.

Of course I didn't know I was about to have one, otherwise I may have taken some action to prevent it (although as you will discover later I had been in discussion with my doctor about some health complications) but I thought the experts that intervened at the hospital where I was treated might have a clue.

I was told that the chances of another heart attack within 5 years were quite high.

But there was no intention from the hospital or my GP to investigate the cause of my heart disease, just a protocol to treat me.

I found the jargon and terminology used on my hospital release paperwork, and in conversation with doctors, was difficult to understand and I was left feeling scared and confused, wanting desperately to know why I had so nearly died, but feeling that I had no idea how to prevent another heart attack from happening.

I couldn't stop smoking, as I didn't smoke.

I wasn't diabetic.

I couldn't lose weight, as I wasn't really overweight (well maybe half a stone).

I could lower my cholesterol a bit more, but it wasn't classed as high.

I could do a bit more exercise, but was already playing tennis for 8 hours a week and exercising at my local gym, so I wasn't exactly sedentary.

I quickly discovered that some of the medications I was prescribed had the potential to be life-limiting, which was really frightening.

Frustrated at the position I found myself in, I decided to learn as much as I could about heart disease.

Since recovering from my heart attack, I have been on a journey to establish what caused it, and what I can do to reverse the damage that I have inadvertently done to my body, to reduce the risk that it will happen again.

What I have discovered along the way is that most of what the general public, and many doctors believe about heart disease is incorrect, and is actually harming the health of their hearts, and their cardiovascular system.

I found that the system for health provision, and the pharmaceutical industry, have in-built problems, which mean its advice should be carefully considered.

I have learned from a growing community of medical experts, that have confronted the disparity between general medical advice, and the real treatments that affect heart disease.

These experts have discovered, through the thorough analysis of research data, and their real-world application, the approaches to tackle chronic modern diseases like CVD, diabetes, Alzheimer's and cancer, and have witnessed the halt and often reversal of some of these chronic diseases in their patients.

They have questioned the status quo, sometimes at great personal and professional sacrifice, to share the information that can prevent heart disease from developing in the healthy, halt the progression of heart disease in the vulnerable, and reverse atherosclerosis (the main protagonist of heart attacks) in those that have already succumbed but survived.

Marcia Agnell - Editor, New England Journal of Medicine, frustrated at the poor advice from the medical establishment wrote this;

"It is simply no longer possible to rely on the judgment of trusted physicians or authoritative medical guidelines. I take no pleasure in this conclusion, which I reached slowly and reluctantly over my two decades as an editor of the New England Journal of Medicine."

Richard Horton - Editor of The Lancet was in accord with her;

"Much of scientific literature, perhaps half, may simply be untrue. Afflicted by studies with small sample sizes, tiny effects, invalid exploratory analyses, and flagrant conflicts of interest, science has taken a turn towards darkness."

The medical community has been very slow to adapt, and accept the facts that confront them where heart disease is concerned.

Doctors are driven by taught protocols that do not improve patient outcomes, and are paid to administer drugs that don't work.

The following statistics relating to heart attacks may surprise you:

- 4 million people die each year across Europe from CVD (45% of all deaths).[2]

---

[2]   https://academic.oup.com/eurheartj/article/37/42/3232/2536403

- 45% of heart attacks are classed as "silent", meaning there is no warning and no prior symptoms.[3]

- Every year around 800,000 Americans suffer a heart attack.[4]

- One person dies every 36 seconds from cardiovascular disease, in the United States alone.[5]

- *Half of all heart attack sufferers have low cholesterol.*[6]

- Estimates have shown that up to 50% of first heart attacks are fatal.[7]

Just take that in for a minute, and digest the statistics above.

Half of all heart attack sufferers were unaware that they had heart disease and they had no obvious risk-factors.

"As many as 50 percent of all cardiac deaths due to disease in the heart's vessels occur in individuals with no prior history or symptoms of heart disease." to quote an article from 2008 in Society of Nuclear Medicine.[8]

3   https://www.health.harvard.edu/heart-health/the-danger-of-silent-heart-attacks

4   https://www.cdc.gov/heartdisease/facts.htm

5   https://www.cdc.gov/heartdisease/facts.htm

6   https://www.health.harvard.edu/heart-health/ask-the-doctor-heart-attack-despite-low-cholesterol

7
    https://www.medicinenet.com/heart_attack_pathology_photo_essay/article.htm

8   https://www.sciencedaily.com/releases/2008/06/080616124938.htm

I am sure you will agree, this is scary!

If, like me, you thought the people likely to have heart attacks were old, overweight, smokers that ate high-fat diets and had really high cholesterol….then you are dead wrong!

We are endlessly told by the media, our GP's and cardiologists that cholesterol is responsible for heart attacks, to the point where many believe this is the only consideration worthy of any measurement.

But the statistics show that 50% of heart attack sufferers have low cholesterol, which means that having high or low cholesterol provides **no predictive benefit at all** for having a heart attack!

Can this be true?

World renowned cardiologist and author of **Wheat Belly**, Dr William Davis is one of many that have analysed the research data and clearly believes so.

"Don't pay any attention to cholesterol. It's ridiculous. It's outdated. It came from the 1950's understanding of heart disease causation." "It is absurd that cholesterol is used as a marker for heart disease....it's a lousy marker." he stated on **The Fat Emperor**, a podcast dedicated to untangling the truth behind the causes of modern chronic disease.

"If all you do is take a statin, lower your cholesterol and take aspirin you have no impact on the progression of the disease.....it's the same as if you do nothing!" He continued….. *"We published this data 20 or so years ago!"*

This is one of the many conundrums that faced me in the spring of 2019, as I searched to uncover why I had just suffered a near fatal heart attack.

Many more myths and mis-information became apparent to me as I studied and learned from experts from all over the world.

I have put much of my accumulated knowledge into this book, in a format that hopefully is explained clearly enough to enable anybody (even my Nan if she were still with us) to understand.

And this is important, because it is not reasonable to expect people not trained in medicine to trawl through medical studies and biological mechanisms, just to learn how to be healthy.

My Nan suffered as her husband, my Grandad, died of a heart attack in his early 60's.

Her son, my Uncle David, also died from a heart attack.

My Nan would not have been able to understand many of the concepts that are discussed in this book, unless they were stated in layman's terms, but she would have wanted to understand the right foods to eat and action to take to protect her family from heart disease.

I hope I have been able to make the concepts that are touched-on in this book clear and devoid of scientific jargon, but whilst also providing enough data, and information on the science behind the conclusions, to provide the fiercest sceptic with convincing evidence of their validity.

In many cases I have added links to articles, books and online resources to support the conclusions I have drawn, and the lifestyle advice that I recommend.

I would, however, always encourage you to think critically, when reading this book as well as any other information relating to health and wellness.

In the age of ever-present media in which we live, it is all too easy to believe everything that is written in a paper, announced on the news and promoted by an "expert".

One of the guiding principles I have employed in my research (as I have often encountered conflicting information or opinions on interpretation of evidence) is to act a little like Hansel and Gretel and follow a path of breadcrumbs back to the source of any irrefutable, trusted data, and look at what the science shows.

It is hard to know what to believe when the opinion of one doctor, or conclusion of one study conflicts with another on the same subject, but when you look back at the raw data from clinical trials, and the evidence from epidemiological studies it is usually easier to separate true facts from biased conclusions.

Sometimes there is no definitive proof of the cause of disease, or the lifestyle choices that can create illness.

In these cases there may not be "hard" evidence from trials, but many different pieces of corollary information, that lead to a fairly certain likely explanation.

My motto is always to try to keep an open mind until one side or the other provides proof (preferably multiple times) of their view. Then I can feel confident that, as unlikely as it might seem sometimes when swimming against the tide of public opinion, I am on the right track.

Some of what you will learn in this book may be hard for you to believe. It may seem contrary to your fundamental understanding about what creates good health. It may be contrary to the advice from your doctor on how to treat or prevent heart disease. It will certainly be at odds with the general media in most cases.

If this is the case, I urge you to read on, to learn more and to delve deeper.

Do not let your pre-conceptions, or your doctors protocols, or poor journalism prevent you from learning what you need to know in order to regain your health.

When you have cause to question the conclusions I draw (and I am sure you will in some cases) it may help to remember that I am a person with heart disease, and at a significant risk of a recurrent heart attack, and everything that I conclude in the book is advice that I take myself, and practice in my life.

The only bias I come to this project with, is that I want the best outcome for my health.

In turn, I hope this is likely to create the best outcomes for the health of those who read this book, that may also be at risk of heart disease.

If you like, think of it as me literally betting my life on the advice contained in Use Your Head, Heal Your Heart!

If having read this book, you feel that its conclusions are at odds with the medical advice that you have been given, then use the information contained herein to question your doctors.

Hold them to account. Have them justify and prove their advice, and the efficacy and safety of any medical interventions they prescribe for you.

HOW TO READ THIS BOOK

In order to make this book easy to navigate it is split into 4 sections: My Story, The Truth About What Causes Heart Disease, Who Is At Risk? & What Can You Do To Prevent Heart Disease or Minimise Risk?

My Story - Feel free to skip this section if you can't wait to dive straight into the learning.

I added my story to provide some context as to how even the people that don't seem likely to suffer from heart disease may actually be in a high-risk group.

One of the biggest challenges with trying to prevent heart disease is that most people don't take the time to learn about it until they already have quite a well developed problem (or are lucky enough to survive a heart attack themselves).

If more people were able to understand their risk earlier, and take action *before* they have symptoms, more would avoid premature death.

Reading about my journey, my life before heart disease and my experience afterwards, might just be the catalyst for you or your loved ones to get tested for the right risk factors early.

My hope is that you have no risk, but that if you do discover an underlying problem early enough, that you can treat it and prevent a life-ending outcome.

The Truth About What Causes Heart Disease - This section explains a little about the history of heart disease, why we hold on to many incorrect beliefs around the causes of heart disease and why the medical community that is supposed to help prevent heart disease often does more harm than good, following out-dated and incorrect guidelines for risk and treatment.

Who Is At Risk? - This section aims to help you to understand your own risk profile, and will explain which tests can provide information to predict heart disease and which don't (with some surprising conclusions).

It will also help you with resources on where you can obtain the information that you won't be able to get from your GP, about your real heart disease risk, and the metrics that you should be focussed on when measuring your progress.

What Can You Do To Prevent Heart Disease or Minimise Risk? - This last section explains what you can do to make a positive impact on any negative risk factors that you uncover from your tests.

I will explain some of the lifestyle, environmental and medical interventions that will help you to address each area that is a problem for you specifically.

I will also provide a system called C.R.A.S.H. which will explain how you might manage the changes in your lifestyle more easily, and adapt better to form some habits that will reduce your CVD risk significantly.

In each section there will be a number of chapters.

I will start each chapter with a short conclusion of the findings for that specific topic, to provide a quick and easy overview.

This, if you like, is the explanation that my Nan would understand.

After this I will go into a little more of the detail, by way of an explanation of how that conclusion was reached, for those that want to understand the concepts and background a little better.

There will be links to references and articles for those that would like a deeper dive into some of the scientific data and clinical trials that have led to the conclusions.

Lastly, there is a summary of the book and links to further reading that I have created to help you on your journey of recovery from heart disease, or to help you live a lifestyle that minimises the risk of you ever suffering from CVD in the first place.

I will also update information on my blog site www.UYHH-YHblog.com.

Thank you for reading this book, and for opening your mind to its contents.

I hope you find it valuable, and I wish you a healthy and well-lived life.

PART 1: MY STORY

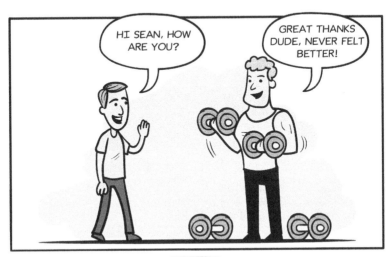

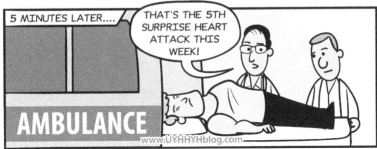

On 17th March 2019 I suffered a heart attack.

- I was 51 years old

- My cholesterol was low/normal

- I hadn't ever smoked

- I wasn't diabetic

- I didn't take drugs

- I weighed 13 stone at 5 ft 9 inches tall, average build (22% body fat)

- I played tennis regularly, and felt fairly fit.

I avoided fat, have no sugar in my tea or coffee, ate plenty of chicken and fish, consumed the odd protein shake after the gym…..just a pretty average guy.

I thought I lived a normal life, and didn't have any reason to feel particularly vulnerable to heart disease.

How could this happen to me?

What was I doing that was so wrong?

Was I so different from other people?

MY HISTORY

I was health conscious and athletic from an early age.

I walked to school, played football before classes and at break-time and would play squash or tennis after school if I got the chance to.

When I got a little older, I took an interest in weight training, and by the time I left school I had decided to take a career in sport, studying sports studies at Farnborough College of Technology, as well as putting myself through separate coaching awards for football, resistance training, swimming, badminton, table-tennis, trampolining, etc.

My first job was as a weight training instructor at Guildford Sports Centre, in their Health & Fitness club called Seagulls.

In this role, before switching to a more financially rewarding career in IT, I took a keen interest in nutrition and worked alongside 3 competing bodybuilders and a British champion powerlifter. I had a 29 inch waist a 40 inch chest and about 9% body fat, weighing just under 12 stone.

I played football to good club standard, and had been captain of the Bracknell Town U19 football team.

I was what most people would refer to as "sporty".

Growing up our family didn't eat too badly either. Or rather we didn't think so.

Through my school years I mainly lived on cereal (sometimes 5 bowls a day) along with school meals which were pretty healthy, baked beans on toast in the evenings and the odd meat-based dish on a Sunday. I was so active I was always very slim, despite eating quite a lot of food.

I distinctly remember the time in the early 1980's when eating fat started to become "demonised", because we were one of the families that switched from butter to margarine, and bought skimmed milk from the supermarket instead of the nice full-fat milk the milkman used to deliver in bottle to the door. My Mum wanted the best for us.

My cereal tasted watery with the tasteless skimmed milk poured all over it, and it almost put me off tea altogether, but as a health-conscious kid I accepted the changes as positive, and we all eventually got used to the taste of these new additions, as the western world adapted to consuming "vegetable oils" instead of dairy produce.

I particularly became so obsessed with avoiding fat that I used to cut it off anything that was ever served up to me…..considering it to be "poison", as was the mantra of the time, and I began to really dislike the taste. I never ate the skin of any chicken dish, removed the rind from bacon and positively never ate steak! (We couldn't afford steak anyway).

When I reached 18 the world of pubs was open to me, but I didn't really drink, and was known as the guy that couldn't finish one pint of beer. I would be pretty much drunk if I ever did.

As I got older and worked my way up into more senior roles for IT companies I did less and less sport, and started a family.

The pressures of work grew, I worked long hours. To be the best dad I could, I would rush home after 5.30 to spend as much time with my young family as possible, and then re-acquaint myself with the computer into the early hours of the morning to catch-up on work that I had missed.

I became a poor sleeper, was in a constant state of stress (although at the time I thought I was coping with it rather well) and was very bad at asking for help. I drank wine more regularly with meals, could afford more take-aways and had less time…so my eating habits slipped into eating more processed food.

To the outside world though, I still looked pretty fit, I could beat most friends at squash and compete at 5-a-side football, so I considered that I was pretty "lucky" to be able to stay in good shape without really putting much effort in.

I did put on some weight in my thirties, and had a new normal weight of nearer to 13 stone than 12 stone.

I guess it was into my forties that things started to become more challenging for me physically.

I went through a stressful divorce, and I really missed seeing my children every day.

After selling part of the company where I was a shareholder, we went through a challenging phase where the new investors sought a conflict with the business founders. This became quite toxic and was finally concluded a few years later when we sold the business, after a lot of stress.

Stressors continued, and culminated in my late forties through some difficult work challenges, and my poor coping mechanisms.

At this time I had noticed, whilst engaged in a work-related challenge, that the conflict had started to make my heart race, and I felt what I now recognise to be anxiety, and an early warning sign that all was not well with me.

This happened about the time that my father starting to suffer badly with vascular dementia, having had a stroke some years earlier.

I went to live with my father for a little over a year, helping him to receive diagnosis and trying to obtain more support.

This proved extremely tiring and stressful on top of everything else that was happening to me, as his condition worsened, and his grasp of reality loosened.

I started to develop a bit of a "victim mentality", and noticed that I wasn't coping as well as I had done with stressors in the past. I started to wonder why so many bad things were happening to me. My mindset was quite negative.

In the midst of all of this, a good friend of mine that had emigrated to the US committed suicide. He was 48.

In September 2018, another close friend of mine, fresh from a week away with me and a few others, was diagnosed with Cancer. On Christmas Day that same year, he passed away, with a few close friends and family members at his bedside.

Three weeks later my father died in January 2019.

After years of not really looking after myself, in the few years prior to my heart attack I had been through a lot of stress, but still I hadn't considered myself to be at risk of heart disease.

Maybe that seems a bit stupid, but outwardly I looked healthy.

I thought my life seemed quite normal, not much different to others, probably healthier than most.

I had noticed one or two times in the year before my heart attack, that when I had been anxious, or when I was exerting myself during tennis matches, I had a tight pressing sensation in my sternum (the middle of my chest).

This happened a couple of times before I mentioned it to my partner Julie.

"Blimey…I am getting pains in my chest. I had better have a lie down, I think I might be having a heart attack!" I joked!

I laughed.

She didn't.

THE REALISATION

Julie convinced me to go and see my GP and explain what had happened.

My conversations with my doctor are paraphrased here, but this is essentially how I remember them.

He ran a standard blood test, looked at the profile and said that it was nothing to worry about. ***"It definitely isn't heart related"*** he said. ***"We can rule that out straight away. You don't smoke, you are fit and your cholesterol levels are really good."***

"I think you should cut back on drinking though, and not eat too many spicy foods as it is likely to be gastro-intestinal or indigestion."

"But it feels like it is in my heart…behind my sternum." I protested.

"Sometimes when it is upper abdominal pain it can feel like it is your chest, but it isn't heart related, so lay off the booze and come back and see me if you don't feel any better after a month or two."

I did drink a bit too much. It was not uncommon for me to have a glass or two of red wine pretty much every night, and on some evenings I would drink a whole bottle.

This frustrating exchange was repeated again with my GP a few months later.

Upon a third visit in 9 months, and after some insistence from me, my GP referred me to a gastro-intestinal consultant to run some specific tests to discover the cause of the chest discomfort.

I remained convinced it was heart-related, the GP remained adamant that it wasn't. He even laughed at my suggestion that it might be.

"When the consultant discovers exactly what the condition is it will put your mind at rest that it isn't your heart." The GP assured me. "You are too young and don't have any of the risk-factors!"

On the 14th March 2019 I visited a gastroenterology specialist, Dr Sassoon Levi, at The Spire Thames Valley private hospital and he ran some comprehensive gastroenterology tests.

At the end of the appointment he gave me the verdict.

"Well, I have some good news and some not so good news." He said.

"The good news is there is absolutely nothing wrong with your whole gastro-intestinal tract and I can't find any problems there at all."

I already guessed the bad news.

"That means it's my chest doesn't it?" I replied.

"I am afraid it does point to that." He concluded.

We both knew that this was a much worse outcome.

He advised me that a CT scan of my heart would confirm what he thought was probably a heart-related issue.

I called my GP and arranged another appointment, so he could refer me to somebody to check-out my heart & lungs and an appointment was planned for a week's time, when I returned from a tennis weekend with the boys and 5 days in Miami watching the Miami Open tennis championship with Julie.

That Friday night I headed off to the tennis weekend in Bournemouth. I played all day Saturday, and felt pretty good. We had a couple of beers and a curry afterwards, and I hit the sack.

The following morning, after a restless night, hot and de-hydrated, I got up and had a full English breakfast and took the short walk with two friends along the promenade at Bournemouth, to where the car was parked. We were planning to go to the tennis centre for another day on-court.

As we approached a short hill I noticed that my left arm started to feel quite tingly and uncomfortable. I shook it off and started clenching my fist to get the blood flowing through it....but it remained uncomfortable anyway.

Then with each step it felt like my legs were filling with lead. Each step got heavier until I realised that I couldn't....or wouldn't dare, take another step forward.

My friends looked behind to see what was holding me up. I smiled and they carried on up the hill. I took two more tentative steps. Then stopped again. "I can't be having a heart attack!" I thought.

But somewhere in my head I was recalling information deep in my sub-conscious;

"If you have tingling down your arm it is a sign that you are having a heart attack!"......"If you feel a shortening of breath for no reason it may be lack of oxygen to the heart."

"Are you OK!?" One of my friends shouted back…….."Yeah, just coming!" I replied.

"Why is it I can't just tell them I am having a heart attack!?" I admonished myself. "For God's sake!…..surely I would rather be embarrassed than collapse in an attempt to hide what's happening?"

Still I said nothing.

I kept hearing my doctor's voice telling me there was no way I had a heart condition.

I kept thinking everybody would think I was a drama-queen if I mentioned it. They would suspect my predicament was the inevitable consequence of a hangover from a night of beer and spend the rest of the day taking the piss out of me.

Slowly, I made my way to the top of the hill. I tried to control my breathing as much as possible and relax my arms and neck.

My left arm was now in a lot of discomfort from the shoulder to my hand.

9

I made it to the car, and sat in the back seat. I closed my eyes, kept very still and tried to meditate….hoping I could "will" the symptoms away….and after 20 minutes in the car they did start to subside.

When we arrived at the tennis centre, I told the boys that I would sit out the first game as I was feeling a bit hungover. We had to walk a really long and convoluted route through changing rooms, past squash courts, up some steps behind a bar, down some stairs and there were the tennis courts right at the back of the club. All the courts were empty. It took about 10 minutes to even find the courts.

As I watched them play I started to feel silly for worrying. Maybe it was just indigestion and a hangover. At this point I didn't know that a night of dehydration from a few beers, and then a full stomach from breakfast, was enough of a stress on the heart of somebody with a blocked artery to trigger a problem on an uphill walk. But it clearly was.

Feeling daft, and not changed for tennis, I wanted to test myself to see if I had imagined what had passed before, so I asked one of the other chaps to have a gentle "hit" with me on one of the empty side courts. "I won't run for much but let's just hit back to each other" I said to him.

A handful of swings later, lunging for a ball out of my reach, I realised what a bad idea this was. I stopped dead in my tracks. I needed to lie down. I edged to the side of the court….loosened my top and lay flat on my back breathing really slowly. The guys in the match looked over. "You bloody attention-seeker….what's wrong now!?" One shouted over. After a few minutes of no response, they stopped the game and came over to see me.

"What is it!?" They now sounded very concerned, and again I felt guilty and overly-dramatic. "I just don't feel too good." I said. "If anybody fancies leaving for home early then I wouldn't mind heading back."

Dave, who lived close to me, agreed to drive the 100 or so miles back to Beaconsfield from Bournemouth, and off we set.

I didn't risk telling him what I feared had happened in case he took me straight to the local hospital. I texted my friend Mike, who is a GP and explained what had happened.

"Get straight to the nearest hospital NOW!" He implored me.

"I am heading back home and will go to the local hospital when I get there." I replied.

"No!" He insisted. "Turn the car around and get to the nearest hospital right now!"

I couldn't face being so far from home, and felt that I could just keep still and control my breathing in the car and I would be OK for the 90 minute drive back.

I told Mike that I would take his advice, but I didn't. We kept on heading for home.

In retrospect this was totally DUMB! And I implore you, if faced with any signs or symptoms like this please just call an ambulance. I would do if this ever happened again.

I got away with this stupid behaviour.

I sent a message to my partner Julie.

"I will be home in about an hour or so" I wrote "can you take me to the hospital as soon as I get there. Nothing too serious, but we will need to be ready to leave straight away."

God knows what she thought, but she was ready and waiting as we arrived.

I thanked Dave for the lift, keeping him in the dark about what was happening. I think he thought I had a really bad hangover.

When we finally arrived at the hospital 2 hours later, I was sent in for a blood test to see if I had elevated levels of a protein called troponin in my blood. The presence of significant levels of troponin are an indication that there has been myocardial necrosis (heart muscle death) from an infarction. (heart attack to you and me).

I was due to fly to Miami the following day with Julie and two friends. We had been looking forward to a week on holiday, watching the ATP tennis event there, and playing a bit of tennis too.

As we waited an hour or so for the blood test results in the hospital I chatted with the cardiologist.

"Do you think I will be able to fly to Miami tomorrow?" I asked. Looking back it seems so ridiculous that I even asked, but I still couldn't quite believe that this had happened to me. It felt like a figment of my imagination.

"If you have had a heart attack you won't be going anywhere!" Came the reply.

I looked at Julie.

"I don't feel too bad now….maybe it was nothing. I feel like such an idiot!"

"Look if the results are under 0.4" the consultant continued "then we will let you go home…but if they are over that figure we will keep you in and have a look at you tomorrow from the inside and see if there is any heart disease."

The test results came back. 0.42! So close!

"That's not that bad. That's pretty close to 0.4. Do you reckon I can go?" I pleaded.

"Sorry. Anything over 0.4 we have to keep you in. Looks like you may have had a little heart attack!"

THE FINDINGS

The next day I was visited by another cardiologist with a team of trainee cardiology students. He asked me a few questions and then let me know that in an hour or so I would be sent to theatre for the surgeons to put a camera into my veins and along with an ultrasound they would have a look at what the picture was from the inside.

If there were any signs of atherosclerosis (thickening of the arterial wall) they would be really clear, and they could insert a stent (a small tubular mesh that expands within the artery to increase blood flow) immediately to clear any blockages.

If the disease was severe, they would need to schedule me in for heart bypass surgery.

"Just read this form and sign it giving us consent to insert a stent if we see a blockage." He handed me a disclaimer that explained everything.

All I remember reading was.

Risks for this procedure:

- damage to the artery where the sheath was inserted

- allergic reaction to the contrast agent used during the procedure

- damage to an artery in the heart

- excessive bleeding requiring a blood transfusion

- ***heart attack, stroke or death***

I was going to be awake and watching whilst this was happening and I had no phone, so I couldn't tell any friends or family that the test might also become a potentially dangerous surgical procedure.

I had this sinking feeling that I was never going to see my children or Julie again.

I was petrified.

When I arrived at theatre the two surgeons seemed very casual. A little local anaesthetic in my arm and then they made and incision and started threading the camera into my veins up towards my heart.

"F*@k! That hurts!" I flinched.

"You shouldn't feel that." One said.

"Well I bloody can...Jesus!"

They tried to pull the camera out but it was clearly stuck.

"Wow...you must have tiny veins." One remarked as they tugged and tugged and my arm was being wrenched upwards.

"Bloody Hell!!!" I shouted again.

They finally removed the camera.

NB. I later learned from the consultant during a run-through of the video of the operation that I have a dog-leg turn in the veins in my arm, and the camera had taken a wrong turn from the main vein to a much smaller one.

"Better go in at the groin." They decided, and the process started again.

Once in, it was intriguing to see what they could see on the screen....but I felt sick and worried at the thought that I could have a re-action, leading to a heart attack at any moment.

"Ah here we go." said one of the surgeons, and proceeded to talk me through the whole procedure while I watched on the screen, as he inserted a stent beautifully.

"So did I have a blockage then!?" I half confirmed, half asked him, in a queasy state as he cleaned-up after the procedure, and the nurse tried to stem the blood-flow from the insertion point.

"Yes...you can see here that this was the blood flow through your LAD before the operation." He pointed to the screen as he played back a recording of the procedure he had just performed.

I saw the liquid pump towards the heart in a wave and then turn to a trickle at a juncture before it reached its destination.

"And here is the same thing after the stent."

Wow what a difference! The blood pumped in the same way, but where before it has trickled through a blockage it just kept on flowing beautifully!

Amazing!

"Thank you so much!" I said with a trembly, emotional voice, conscious of how inadequate saying "thank you" is when someone has basically performed life-saving surgery on you with no complications.

"No problem. That should give you a new lease of life. You will feel 18 again after this."

"Really!?" I laughed through teary eyes.

"Oh yes!" He replied. "Your LAD was 90% blocked."

"Bloody Hell...really!" I was shocked. "That sounds pretty bad!"

"You were lucky, your heart is pretty strong and it seems there was very little damage to the heart muscle. Do you play any sport!?"

"Yes a bit of tennis." I replied. "In fact I was on a tennis holiday when this happened, and I was going to be on a tennis holiday today."

"Well you got away with quite a small amount of damage, but it's a good job you didn't go on your holiday." he replied. "The LAD (Left

Artery Descending) is known as the 'widowmaker'! They call it that because it does more work than the other two arteries. When it is blocked, you have such a short amount of time to get assistance before a heart attack, that for most people there isn't enough time to be saved. Your next game of tennis would probably have been your last one...if you know what I mean."

So, now you know how a chap, with no obvious risk factors and in relatively good health can have a near fatal heart attack at 51.

I was so perplexed by my condition, and so shocked by the contradictory information that I received before, and after my heart attack, that I felt compelled to learn more, and understand the facts behind heart disease.

It was then that I started to discover the myths about cholesterol and saturated fat.

Part 2: The Truth About What Causes Heart Disease

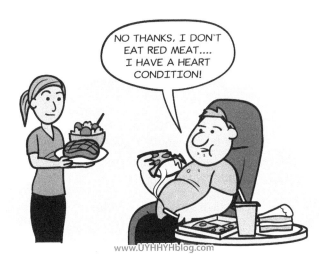

How is it that we can get to a stage where a disease that progresses very slowly, over a long period of time, can creep-up on us in the way my heart attack did, with nobody spotting the problem along the way?

I didn't have a main artery 90% blocked overnight, it must have taken years to develop that level of atherosclerosis.

Why did it take me three attempts to try to convince my GP that I had a problem with my heart, and even then he did not accept that I did?

Do we really know what causes heart disease, if it can't be discovered until it is too late for most people?

It seems it can be discovered if one looks for the right clues. The problem seems to be that our doctors often look at irrelevant information, presuming those results can provide us with a perfect bill of health.

If doctors really are looking at the wrong indicators, does that also mean that the advice to moderate those indicators is wrong?

This would mean the advice that we are given to keep our hearts healthy is also wrong, and we are living with false beliefs about the causes of heart disease.

OK, get ready to have your perspective completely turned on its head.

If you are like me, and most of the people I come across, and you have spent most of your life thinking that you know roughly which foods are good for human health and which foods are bad, you may be about to have your beliefs challenged.

This is especially true when it comes to heart health and the development of heart disease.

Most of what you believe to be true about saturated fat and heart health is completely wrong!

This isn't really your fault.

You, like me and millions of the rest of the Western world have been taken for a bit of a ride by some bad science and flawed data that was then manipulated by ambitious, political individuals, and then perpetuated and funded by huge sums of money from the sugar, agriculture, FMCG and pharmaceutical interests in the USA, whilst they protected their assets.

It all started in the 1950's.

But we will deal with that in a later chapter.

WHAT DOESN'T CAUSES HEART DISEASE

Nan's Chapter Summary: *For many years we have believed that saturated fat creates heart disease. Many studies have been undertaken to try to establish if this is actually true. When all of these studies have been analysed, it has become clear that researchers can find no evidence that saturated fat, or even cholesterol cause heart disease. In fact in some studies eating more saturated fat helped to decrease strokes.*

We have been wrong to believe that high saturated fat and high cholesterol in our diets contribute to heart disease!

SATURATED FAT!

Difficult as this will be to digest for most people (excuse the pun)......

Saturated fat doesn't cause heart disease!

This has been demonstrated in medical research many, many times, but for some reason this is not widely shared with the general public.

For example, one 2014 review of 32 other medical studies[1] that included 659,298 people found

"No significant association between saturated fat intake and heart disease."

There's more, a meta-analysis of prospective epidemiologic studies in 2010 [2] followed-up 347,747 subjects over up to 23 years and showed that there is;

"No significant evidence for concluding that dietary saturated fat is associated with an increased risk of CHD or CVD."

and that..

"further research doesn't show a significant association between saturated fat intake and all-cause mortality or stroke."

---

[1] https://pubmed.ncbi.nlm.nih.gov/24723079/

[2] https://pubmed.ncbi.nlm.nih.gov/20071648/

20

Another systematic review and meta-analysis from 2015 [3] showed that;

"Saturated fats are not associated with all cause mortality, CVD, CHD, ischaemic stroke, or type 2 diabetes."

Confused!?

It would seem from the medical communities own research, covering many other clinical trials and studies, covering hundreds and thousands of subjects, that they all conclude the same thing......that saturated fat has no association with CHD, CVD, strokes, diabetes or "all cause" mortality.

Why do we have the mistaken belief that it does then?

Food consumption and the actual statistics of cardiovascular diseases: [4] is an epidemiological comparison of 42 European countries based on the average consumption of 62 different foods.

The aim of this study was to identify the main nutritional factors that were related to the prevalence of cardiovascular diseases in Europe, based on a comparison of international statistics.

This is what the researchers discovered:

"Remarkably, the relationship of raised cholesterol with CVD risk is always negative, especially in the case of total CVD mortality."

"The most significant dietary correlate of low CVD risk was high total fat and animal protein consumption."

---

3   https://pubmed.ncbi.nlm.nih.gov/26268692/

4   https://www.ncbi.nlm.nih.gov/pmc/articles/PMC5040825/

What!?

Just to repeat that last conclusion…..*high total fat and animal protein correlates with LOW CVD risk!*

They went on.

"Our results do not support the association between CVD and saturated fat, which is still contained in official dietary guidelines. Instead, they agree with data accumulated from recent studies that link CVD risk with the high glycemic index/load of carbohydrate-based diets."

"In the absence of any scientific evidence connecting saturated fat with CVD, these findings show that current dietary recommendations regarding CVD should be seriously reconsidered."

At this point I am trying not to overwhelm you with every piece of scientific evidence that reaches this conclusion, because there is lots of it, but I hope I have added a few examples to help to make the point that from a scientific perspective, saturated fat does not cause heart disease.

The reason saturated fat got dragged into the debate about what causes heart disease, is because of the associated between saturated fat consumption and cholesterol levels.

Your cholesterol levels are largely genetic….If you eat less your body produces more and if you eat more your body produces less.

However, there is some affect on your cholesterol levels (circa plus or minus 15%) that you can achieve, based on your diet.

If you eat more saturated fat you can slightly increase your cholesterol levels, and in turn you can increase the type of cholesterol profile that you have. (You improve it actually).

If you eat less saturated fat and replace it with certain plant sterols, you can slightly decrease your cholesterol levels by a similar degree. (Which evidence shows to be harmful).

Vegans and vegetarians often proudly (and mistakenly) proclaim the benefits of plant sterols effects on reducing cholesterol, when in fact this is not good for your heart health according to scientific studies.

In actual fact, this is one of the reasons (and there are a few more) that an exclusively plant-based diet can work *against* your heart health to some degree.

Because it has been erroneously theorised, historically, that higher cholesterol causes heart disease, it was then an automatic belief that saturated fat (as a consequence of increasing cholesterol) was a protagonist of heart disease, and should be removed from the diet.

But once you understand that cholesterol is NOT the cause of heart disease, then there is no basis for avoiding saturated fat, and this is the reason why, when anybody tries to make the connection between saturated fat and heart disease in a scientific trial (and a lot of pharmaceutical companies that make money from cholesterol-lowering drugs have tried many times to do this) the results prove to be disappointing, as no relationship has been shown.

The National Institute of Health (NIH) eventually spent between $500,000 and $1 billion testing the hypothesis that a low-fat diet would prevent chronic disease in women, and bestow on them a longer life.

The **Women's Health Initiative** trial at and estimated circa $725 million cost, was the largest randomised clinical controlled trial of the low-fat diet ever undertaken.

49,000 post-menopausal women were given a low-fat diet and assigned intervention groups to hormone replacement therapy and calcium and vitamin D supplementation.

More than 20,000 women in the low-fat diet group were instructed to cut back on meat, eggs, butter, cream, salad dressings and other fatty foods.

The low-fat diet had been the official recommended diet of the American Heart Association for more than 30 years at this point.

This study was the first to establish whether this diet actually works.

The women in the study successfully reduced their overall fat from 37% to 29% of calories and their saturated fat was reduced from 12% to 9% of calories.

They met their targets to achieve this, but after a decade of following this diet they were no less likely than the control group to contract breast cancer colorectal cancer ovarian cancer endometrial cancer/or even heart disease.

Despite decades of clinical trials and epidemiological studies, and literally billions of dollars of expenditure, there is no evidence anywhere that demonstrates that saturated fat intake causes heart disease!

Saturated Fats and Health: A Reassessment and Proposal for Food-Based Recommendations [5] is a 2020 review which stated;

"Most recent meta-analyses of randomised trials and observational studies found no beneficial effects of reducing saturated fat intake on cardiovascular disease (CVD) and total mortality, and instead found protective effects against stroke."

---

[5]   https://pubmed.ncbi.nlm.nih.gov/32562735/

Part 2: The Truth About What Causes Heart Disease

CHOLESTEROL!

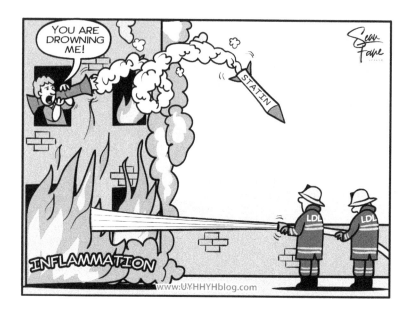

*"Choose a job. Choose a career. Choose a family. Choose a f******g big television. Choose washing machines, cars, compact disc players and electrical tin openers. Choose good health, low cholesterol, and dental insurance. Choose fixed interest mortgage repayments".*

Since long before the sage advice delivered by Renton from the opening lines of the 1996 film Trainspotting, about 3 Edinburgh lads and their disregard of all things they knew to be sensible in favour of the ecstatic highs of heroin, lowering cholesterol has been considered a universal imperative for good health.

We all know that high cholesterol causes heart disease....right?

You can ask 100 people what causes a heart attack and it is likely that 99 of them will respond with "high cholesterol".

Only its not true!

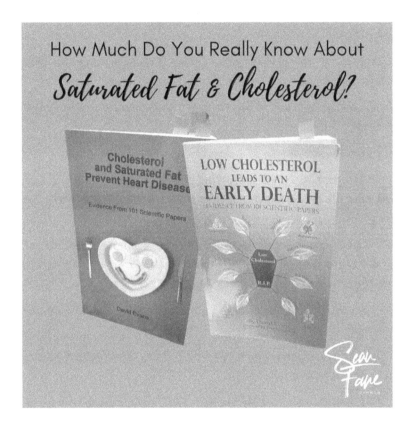

Cholesterol doesn't cause heart disease!

Back to one of the studies I referred to in the section above on saturated fat, which covered the 62 foods consumed across 42 countries.

They had more to say on the relationship between saturated fat and cholesterol.

"The results of our study show that animal fat (and especially its combination with animal protein) is a very strong predictor of raised cholesterol levels. This is in accordance with the meta-analyses of clinical trials, which show that saturated animal fat is the major trigger of raised cholesterol."

Ah, so they say that saturated fat doesn't cause heart disease, but it can raise cholesterol.

So you might presume that they go on to conclude that this might increase CVD then?

No, they continued..

"Interestingly, the relationship between raised cholesterol and CVD indicators in the present study is always negative."

"The negative relationship between raised cholesterol and CVD may seem counterintuitive, but it is not at variance with the available evidence."

Even your GP probably hasn't got this message yet (although they are starting to catch-on).

It's pretty hard to get your head around this after years of believing it to be an uncontested fact of life.

Not only do most people not know that high cholesterol is not a predictor of heart disease, but most are totally unwilling to comprehend or even listen to anybody that challenges this belief.

The "Good" cholesterol often referred to in most news articles and media channels and conversations with your friends and family would be HDL (High Density Lipoprotein) and the "bad" cholesterol would be LDL (Low Density Lipoprotein).

This too is not an accurate picture of the facts.

NB. NEVER get your health advice from the mainstream media....they often perform terrible research and follow flawed governmental guidelines and know very little about most health related science.

WHAT IS CHOLESTEROL?

Nan's Chapter Summary: *Cholesterol is the name for groups of molecules that are produced by our liver. They travel to areas of damage, or bacterial infection, and deliver the resources needed to repair the damage or fight-off the bacteria.*

Without cholesterol we would die.

Cholesterol is important for brain health and memory, hormone production, and the absorption of vitamin D from the sun.

It is also responsible for fighting-off roughly 70% of the things that attack our bodies, like bacteria and viruses, which means as we get older and more vulnerable to illness, it is more important than ever that our cholesterol levels are maintained at a healthy level.

Our cholesterol levels are actually determined for us by our genetics, and our body keeps our own individual level of cholesterol pretty-much the same all the time.

We can get some cholesterol from our diets, but if we eat more cholesterol it doesn't mean our level increases, it just means our liver produces less to maintain our level. If we eat less cholesterol our liver just produces more. So eating cholesterol in foods makes no difference to our cholesterol levels.

We can, however, increase our cholesterol levels slightly, and improve the size of cholesterol molecules we have, by having a diet rich in saturated fats.

The size of our cholesterol molecules can be a factor in whether they are able to become damaged by infections or bacteria.

Sometimes when the cholesterol is healing a damaged area of the body, like an artery wall for example, other infections or bacteria in our blood can react with the cholesterol molecule. When this happens the area can become inflamed, and sometimes will form a scar. These scars can become thick enough, over time, to block some of the blood from travelling through the arteries. This is one of the main causes of heart attacks.

Let me first explain what LDL and HDL are, and you will understand why they are important for our bodies. I will try to keep it simple.

Cholesterol is the name given to a molecule that makes-up 30% of the cells of all mammals.

It is the essential structural component of the cell membrane, so the 37 trillion (give or take a trillion or so) cells in your body all need cholesterol.

Without it you would have no cell structure at all…..and you would die.

Cholesterol is essential for neuro-transmitter function. The ability for cells to communicate.

According to Chris Masterjohn, a doctor with a PhD in Nutritional Sciences from the University of Connecticut who runs a blog called The Daily Lipid and has published a class and supporting book called *Vitamins & Minerals 101*;

"Cholesterol is found in every cell of your body. It helps to maintain the integrity of the membranes and plays a role in facilitating signalling. It keeps your membranes from turning to mush!"[6]

Cholesterol is not soluble in water, so to enable it to flow through the blood (which is water-based) it is transported (from the liver where most of it is created) in lipoproteins, which act as a water-soluble taxi

---

6   https://chris-masterjohn-phd.myshopify.com/products/vitamins-and-minerals-101-pre-order

service delivering the cholesterol to the cells that require it…hence the need for LDL, HDL and the rest of the lipoprotein taxis. The density relates to their direction of travel to and from the liver.

There is one particular area of the body, that needs a lot of cholesterol…the brain.

In the article *The Effects of Cholesterol on Learning & Memory*[7] it was stated;

"Cholesterol is ubiquitous in the central nervous system and vital to normal brain function including; signalling, synaptic plasticity, learning & memory. Cholesterol is so important to brain function that it is generated independently of cholesterol metabolism in the rest of the body and is sequestered by the blood brain barrier."

Although the brain represents only 2% of our total body weight, it contains 20% of the body's cholesterol.

"Synapses, the magical areas where communication between brain cells take place, are lined by cholesterol-rich membranes responsible for passing neurotransmitters like serotonin, GABA, and dopamine back and forth."

"Cholesterol also helps guide developing nerve endings to their destinations."

"If the brain is too low in cholesterol, it's membranes, synapses, myelin and lipid rafts can't form or function

---

[7]

https://www.sciencedirect.com/science/article/abs/pii/S0149763410000941

properly, bringing all brain activity, including mood regulation, learning, and memory to a screeching halt. "Says Georgia Ede, MD in *Psychology Today*'s online blog.

Sounds pretty important then this cholesterol stuff.

Your brain has something called the blood-brain barrier.

The blood–brain barrier is a highly-selective, semipermeable border of endothelial cells (which act like a nightclub doorman) that prevent anything in the circulating blood from non-selectively crossing into the fluid of the central nervous system where neurons reside.

So in order to get all the cholesterol it needs without relying on blood-flow, the brain produces its own cholesterol.

Like the liver, brain cells depend on a substance called **HMG-CoA reductase** to produce cholesterol.

This is interesting because there are products that stop the body from producing **HMG-CoA reductase** which is a monumentally daft thing to do based on its importance to your brain.

As you can imagine, drugs that do this have some pretty dire consequences for brain performance, mood, depression, memory, concentration, and can even lead to Alzheimer's and dementia.

Rather than call them **HMG-CoA reductase inhibitors** (which is their medical term but I can only presume wasn't thought to be a terribly "catchy" name) the medical community decided to refer to these products by the, much easier to remember, name of statins.

Now you know why statins have been shown to have terrible consequences for brain health.

In his book **Lipitor - Thief Of Memory** Dr Duane Graveline, former astronaut, aerospace medical research scientist, flight surgeon, and family doctor describes a "scary" ordeal that he went through.

He lost both short-term and retrograde memory, and was finally diagnosed as having transient global amnesia (TGA), as a result of taking statins, and his book recounts his journey back to health after he stopped taking the statins.

Anyway, back to cholesterol and their lipoprotein taxi services, LDL and HDL.

The job of these lipoproteins is just to transport cholesterol through the body, via the blood, and deposit it where it is needed for cellular repair, and then transport any unused cholesterol back to the liver to be recycled.

There are more lipoproteins than just HDL and LDL and they are categorised by their density as they make their way through the body; VLDL (Very Low-Density Lipoproteins), ULDL (Ultra-Low-Density lipoproteins....yes really) and LP(a) (we will talk more about LP(a) later).

They are also categorised by their different particle size, and this has also recently been discovered to play a major role in whether they inadvertently have a greater propensity to become oxidised, which is important. More on this later too.

VLDL's transfer newly created triglycerides and cholesterol out of the liver, to be used in organs and cells around the body. As they lose triglycerides they shrivel down to become LDL.

When a cell in your body needs cholesterol (which it may do to help repair damage) it manufactures an LDL "receptor" and waits for the passing LDL travelling in the blood to attach to it.

Then the LDL delivers the nutrients needed to repair cellular damage.

So each LDL molecule is like a little handy-man flowing through your blood looking for areas of damage and patching them up.

Cholesterol isn't just a handyman though. It is also the foundational material from which many of your hormones are manufactured including:

Aldosterone - which regulates blood pressure

Cortisol - which regulates many functions to elicit a "fight or flight" response

Oestrogen - a female sex hormone

Progesterone - a female sex hormone

Testosterone - a male sex hormone

DHEA - a sex, neural and steroidal hormone

Vitamin D - a pre-hormone used to manufacture other hormones and regulate immune health (it is synthesised in the skin when sunlight meets cholesterol)

As you will learn throughout this book, your hormones are basically the most important chemicals in your body.

They are the things that instruct your body to make the chemical changes needed to adapt and respond to the environment around you, what you eat, what you breathe, how you feel… everything.

When you are too cold your hormones tell your body to warm-up (shiver, re-direct blood, increase metabolism).

When you are short of nutrients…your hormones will tell you to be hungry (yep you don't feel hungry because your stomach is empty, it is your hormones signalling you to eat, whether your stomach is empty or not).

The same when you feel full….you haven't actually exceeded your stomach's ability to store any more food…it is a hormone that tells you that you are full.

Hormones do all this stuff (which you are conscious of) and a whole lot of stuff inside your body that you aren't conscious of. They basically control everything in your body.

Generally the brain makes a signal to ask a gland (or multiple glands) to produce a hormone (or multiple hormones) to fulfil a task to keep you healthy and functioning......all day....every day, based on what your environment throws at you (or what you throw at yourself).

When you look at this list of hormones below some may be recognisable to you.

Oestrogen & Testosterone are well known as the "sex" hormones. If they require cholesterol in order to be synthesised by the body, think of how you might be affected by a reduction or imbalance of these if your cholesterol is too low? Low sex-drive, erectile dysfunction, infertility, depression, hair loss, fat accumulation....these are a few of the implications of sex hormone imbalance.

Vitamin D has several important functions. Perhaps the most vital are regulating the absorption of calcium and phosphorus, and facilitating normal immune system function. Getting a sufficient amount of vitamin D is important for normal growth and development of bones and teeth, as well as improved resistance against certain diseases, bacteria and viruses.

If your body doesn't get enough vitamin D, you're at risk of developing bone abnormalities such as soft bones (osteomalacia) or fragile bones (osteoporosis).

Cross-sectional studies have reported that vitamin D deficiency is associated with increased risk of cardio vascular disease, including hypertension, heart failure, and ischemic heart disease.

It is also critical for good immune function, and helps both reject pathogens and also kill them if they breach your defences...which is why vitamin D has been discovered to be one of the biggest factors impacting survival rates for COVID-19 and other respiratory infections.

Low vitamin D, created by dark winter months (and our subsequent reduced sun exposure) is one of the key factors for why we get respiratory infections in winter (colds, flu, etc) particularly in the Northern Hemisphere.

Aldosterone is synthesised from cholesterol in the adrenal glands. It controls potassium and sodium levels and, by extension, your blood pressure.

So abnormal aldosterone levels may affect your ability to control blood-pressure, which increases your heart disease risk.

DHEA is one of the most abundant circulating steroids in humans and is responsible for many functions relating to hormonal balance, growth and nervous system function.

All of these hormones require cholesterol.

Cholesterol is mostly produced in your liver.

About 80% of your bodies cholesterol is generated in the liver, but cells can also synthesise a small amount themselves if necessary, and we can also get some from our diets.

The liver is a pretty amazing organ.

Think of your liver as your very own chemistry laboratory.

Its job is to use the raw materials that you get from your diet and other substances flowing through your body, filtering out the things you don't need, or converting them into things you do need for good health from any foods you eat.

Here are a few of the main jobs your liver undertakes:

- *Bile Production*: Bile helps you break-down and absorb fats, cholesterol, and some vitamins.

- ***Bilirubin Absorption & Metabolism***: Bilirubin is formed by the breakdown of haemoglobin. The iron released from haemoglobin is stored in the liver or bone marrow and used to make the next generation of blood cells.

- ***Clotting Support***: Vitamin K is necessary for the creation of certain coagulants that help clot the blood. Bile is essential for vitamin K absorption and is created in the liver. If the liver does not produce enough bile, clotting factors cannot be produced.

- ***Carbohydrate Metabolism***: Carbohydrates are stored in the liver, where they are broken down into glucose and siphoned into the bloodstream to maintain normal glucose levels. They are stored as glycogen and released whenever a quick burst of energy is needed.

- ***Vitamin & Mineral Storage***: The liver stores vitamins A, D, E, K, and B12. It keeps significant amounts of these vitamins stocked-up. In some cases, several years' worth of vitamins is held as a backup. The liver stores iron from haemoglobin in the form of ferritin, ready to make new red blood cells. The liver also stores and releases copper.

- ***Protein Metabolism***: Bile helps break down proteins for digestion.

- ***Blood Filtration***: The liver filters and removes compounds from the body, including hormones, such as oestrogen and aldosterone, and compounds from outside the body, including alcohol and other drugs.

- ***Immunological Function***: The liver is part of the mononuclear phagocyte system. It contains high numbers of Kupffer cells that are involved in immune activity. These cells destroy any disease-causing agents that might enter the liver through the gut.

- *Albumin Production*: Albumin is the most common protein in blood serum. It transports fatty acids and steroid hormones to help maintain the correct pressure and prevent the leaking of blood vessels.

- *Angiotensinogen Synthesis*: This hormone raises blood pressure by narrowing the blood vessels when alerted by production of an enzyme called renin in the kidneys.

Arguably one of the most important tasks that your liver undertakes, in addition to these life critical functions, is the production of cholesterol.

There is a rare disease called SLOS (Smith-Lemli-Optitz Syndrome). Those born with SLOS have very low cholesterol due to issues with cholesterol synthesis.

Sadly, they suffer a wide number of challenges including slow growth before and after birth. These challenges are defined at www.rarediseases.org as;

"A small head (microcephaly), mild to moderate mental "retardation" and multiple birth defects (including particular facial features), cleft palate, heart defects, fused second and third toes, extra fingers and toes and underdeveloped genitals in males. This is because their neurones cannot develop properly, due to a lack of cholesterol."

About 25% of those that are born with SLOS will die in early childhood, whilst others can live to adulthood but suffer terribly from the effects of low cholesterol whilst they are alive.

We are often told that there is "good" cholesterol (HDL) and "bad" cholesterol (LDL).

39

So, is there "good" and "bad" cholesterol?

No, is the short answer. It's all good.

We didn't evolve from ancestors over 6 million years, and as our current human species for 200,000 years to create a substance used in every cell, that is "bad" for our health.

A substance manufactured in the liver and with a backup production in the brain, and with the ability for each cell to produce a small amount on its own.

If you don't believe that we are designed to have cholesterol, then you don't believe in evolution as a concept.

Johnny Bowden & Stephen Sinatra had this to say about LDL in their book *The Great Cholesterol Myth*:

"LDL is itself able to inactivate more than 90% of the worst and most toxic bacterial products. Studies have linked low cholesterol to a greater risk for infections."

"LDL does not just neutralise exotoxins. It binds to the bacteria themselves and holds them in place to be attacked and killed by white blood cells." explains Malcolm Kendrick in his book A Statin Nation…and he continued…

"High cholesterol levels get increasingly beneficial as we get older. After the age of about 60, the higher your LDL levels is, the longer you will live, because infections become and increasingly common cause of death as we age."

"A review of 19 large peer-reviewed studies of more than 68,000 deaths, found that low cholesterol predicts a greater risk of dying from respiratory and gastric intestinal diseases."

Hmmmmm respiratory……you mean like COVID-19?

"Another study that followed more than 100,000 healthy individuals in San Francisco, found that those that had low cholesterol at the beginning of the 15 year study were far more likely to be admitted to hospital with infectious diseases."

Still think LDL is "bad"!?

I hope not!

What about HDL…the "good" cholesterol? Isn't this the one that is supposed to help prevent heart disease?

Remember HDL refers to the transporters that take any residual cholesterol **back to the liver** to be re-cycled and processed back into LDL when it is needed.

Thinking of it as uniquely "good" is misleading, however, as it is not something that is independently useful, except in its relationship to clearing utilised LDL for re-cycling.

Dr Malcolm Kendrick again….

"Raising HDL will have no effect on heart disease, as the underlying concept is the finest 100 percent baloney."

"HDL does, however, mop-up "free-cholesterol" in the bloodstream."

HDL does have a, not often mentioned, benefit though as he continues….

"HDL is also an anti-coagulant, and raises the possibility that "good" cholesterol does not provide protection due to any effect on LDL cholesterol. It is because it stops blood clotting."

Low HDL has been linked in trials to an increased risk of heart disease, but that is more to do with the ratios to LDL, because a positive

HDL to LDL ratio means that the transport mechanisms work efficiently to take cholesterol into and out of the blood from the liver.

This has been shown to help "clean-up" the blood, and very low HDL can cause some issues in this respect.

The Framingham Heart Study began in 1948, and is a longitudinal cohort study, a type of epidemiological study that follows a group of individuals over time to determine the natural history of certain diseases, explore the behaviour of those diseases, and identify the factors that might explain their development.

It had an original cohort of 5,209 men and women and has expanded and added generations over the last 72 years.

Much of the now-common knowledge concerning heart disease, such as the effects of diet, exercise, and common medications such as aspirin, is based on this study's analysis.

Here are some of the findings from Framingham over the years that relate to cholesterol.

"People with low HDL (below 35mg/dL) have an 8 times higher rate of heart attacks than those with levels of 65mg/dL and above."

"For each 1% mg/dL drop in cholesterol, there was an 11% increase in coronary and total mortality."

"Half of the people that had heart attacks had cholesterol levels below the "normal" level of 220 mg/dL."

"For men aged 48-57, those with mid-range cholesterol of 183 to 222 mg/dL had a greater risk of heart disease than those with the higher levels of 222 to 261 mg/dL."

William Castelli, a Framingham Heart Study Director, finally admitted in 1992 *"In Framingham the more saturated fat one ate...the lower a persons serum cholesterol...and they weighed the least."*

This highlights that getting a good HDL to LDL ratio, and to keep all the health benefits of high LDL too, one should try to raise HDL if it is very low....NOT lower one's LDL.

And it is in this respect that I have some great news, because pretty much the only way to raise HDL if it is low, also raises LDL a little bit too.

This one dietary intervention, that anybody can do, has the multiple positive outcomes of improving the ratio of HDL & LDL and also improves the particle size of your cholesterol molecules.....and it is achieved by eating something that you have been told for 50 years will kill you..........saturated fat!

I know right!?

No wonder Eskimo's living on nothing but fatty seal blubber for generations had no heart disease!

So this ill-informed notion that HDL and LDL are opposite sides to a coin, with one being "good" and the other "bad" is a misleading belief.

They are both transporters of the same molecule, which is essential to life and good health, but they transport the cargo either *to* or *from* the liver.

Anything you do to reduce your cholesterol, is ultimately damaging to your health.

Once you are released from hospital after a heart attack you will be told quite a lot of daft, contradictory information about cholesterol.

You will be advised to consume less than 200mg of cholesterol per day, regardless of the fact that your liver feels the need to produce more than 10 times that each day to keep you healthy!!

One Salmon fillet....considered ubiquitously as the healthiest food you can consume for you heart, will be a recommended dietary staple......but contains 217.8g of cholesterol (more than your daily recommended allowance).

Find any article or study or trial anywhere that says salmon is bad for your heart. You won't. Every time you read about it it is described as the pinnacle of healthy fish to eat!

For more reading relating to cholesterol and saturated fat, and specifically the evidence of their preventative impact on heart disease and how reducing cholesterol is damaging, I would recommend these two books by David Evans that summarise the scientific research:

Low Cholesterol Leads to an Early Death - Evidence from 101 Scientific Papers.

And

Cholesterol and Saturated Fat Prevent Heart Disease - Evidence from 101 Scientific Papers.

I will leave you with some more prescient advice on LDL from Dr Malcolm Kendrick, at a time when avoiding infections and viruses, and avoiding hospital visits has never been more desirable.

"LDL binds to exotoxins as they are released from bacteria, which protects the endothelium from damage. Because of this, people with higher LDL levels are much less likely to end up in hospital with infections."

The question that now becomes really apparent, after discovering what categorically doesn't cause heart disease, is what *does*?

WHAT CAUSES HEART DISEASE?

Nan's Chapter Summary: Heart attacks are mostly a result of your body responding to damaged artery walls, and creating an accumulation of scar tissue.

You may have some genes that you have inherited that make you more likely to develop problems when you damage your artery walls.

Factors that can make artery wall damage more likely, include things that create hormone imbalances, like too little exercise, not enough exposure to sunshine, stress, poor sleep, damaging relationships and loneliness".

You may also have a lifestyle that creates an environment which causes oxidation in your body, a bit like rust on metal.

Some of the lifestyle factors which can cause this rusting effect include smoking, poor air quality, food high in sugar and starch, vegetable oils.

If you have stayed with me so far, and believe the data, and not the hyperbole from the poorly informed news and media channels, and if you are starting to understand what our flawed education of doctors fails to teach them in medical school, you are probably wondering what does cause a heart attack.

Well, it isn't just one thing.

It is a multi-faceted disease (or collection of diseases) but there are a few simple principles that do generate a very high risk for all of them.

Once you understand the fundamental principles contributing to heart disease, then you may start to understand how various factors can create a cascade of health issues that can lead to a heart attack.

We mentioned hormones earlier….and in essence, the bulk of the challenge of heart disease can be thought of as a hormone imbalance issue, along with some genetic and lifestyle problems to accelerate and exacerbate the problem.

Once certain key hormonal functions start failing in their search for equilibrium, they create a cascade of damage.

Where there is damage, the body seeks to repair it.

When the repair is in the endothelium (the inner lining of an artery wall) the area repaired can become thick and gooey with plaques, and when these plaques narrow the artery diameter, and then rupture and break off, they can create a blockage.

This is a very common form of heart attack and would be written on medical notes afterwards as a myocardial infarction.

The loss of blood flow to your heart will ultimately starve part of your heart of oxygen, and the oxygen-starved muscle cells will soon die, creating a weakened and malfunctioning heart, and possibly also causing an arrhythmia (abnormal beating pattern).

This may, and often does, result in death.

If you are lucky, like me, you will notice the signs of an impending heart attack (or actually feel it starting) and receive treatment to thin your blood, improve your blood pressure, and relieve any blockage before the loss of oxygen to your heart goes past the point of "no return".

Then you are just left with the minor challenge of how you got to this point in the first place and how to prevent it from happening again (which is very common within 5 years off the first heart attack!).

But that's where the many voices of reason, logic and research can help you to find a way back to health.

The best way to prevent heart disease is to have a lifestyle that doesn't create the hormonal imbalances, or inflammation and oxidation in the first place, particularly not in your arteries.

The main causes and their mechanisms are described below.

GENETICS

Our cholesterol level is genetically decided….but some people can have too much or too little.

Familial Hypercholesterolaemia is where a gene predicates that your body will produce very, very high levels of cholesterol.

The effectiveness of cholesterol in fighting infectious diseases, by far the biggest killer of humans before heart disease was "created" by us in the last century, has been known for some time.

"A study done in the Netherlands found that people with FH (familial hypercholesterolaemia) lived longer than anybody else in the nineteenth century." Dr Malcolm Kendrick

FH and Smith-Lemli-Optitz Syndrome are opposite ends of the genetic spectrum.

One is a genetically high cholesterol level and the other is genetically low cholesterol.

In other words, you can't do much about them.

If you visit your GP and they rub their chin and tell you your cholesterol is high, (and they probably will as the government guidelines for "normal" cholesterol are being lowered and lowered year after year) then you need to evaluate whether high means, *a bit higher than their guidelines*, or *really high in the sense of having FH*.

If you do have FH (and only about 1 in 200 people do) then you are more likely to accelerate the advancement of atherosclerosis, but only *if you create the inflammation and oxidation required to start the process*. (This will be explained later when we discuss what does cause heart disease).

If you have FH, any negative lifestyle factors that would otherwise have lead to you experiencing a heart attack at say, 60, might lead to one at a much younger age as you accelerate the build-up of atherosclerotic plaque.

If, however, you reduce your lifestyle risk factors for heart disease (which is what this book aims to teach you to do) then all the surplus LDL that you have circling around in your body will have nothing to repair, and you should avoid heart disease.

In fact if you have FH you are more likely to actually have a relatively disease-free, long life as a consequence of the excess immune-boosting LDL in your system.

You should be very, very careful to avoid inflammation though, and anybody with FH should keep reading through to the C.R.A.S.H. course section of this book and pay close attention to the lifestyle factors that they can positively influence.

PARTICLE SIZE

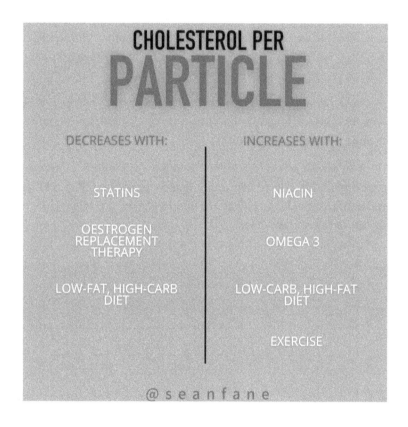

So, should we eat saturated fat?

After all, if there is minimal impact on our cholesterol levels whether we eat saturated fat or not, maybe we might think…..just to be on the safe side….that it is best to avoid saturated fat altogether.

The answer to this is definitely NO!

Quite the opposite!

We already know from what has been covered so far, that cholesterol performs many positive and vital functions in our body, so we should aim to increase our cholesterol (unless you have FH…and then you already have more than enough).

I also mentioned that saturated fat can improve the ratio of HDL to LDL, so that is another reason to eat more.

What hasn't been mentioned yet is the very positive effect that saturated fat has on the particle size of our lipoproteins.

Cholesterol, as I mentioned before consists of a variety of densities of lipoproteins that act as transport vehicles. ULDL, VLDL, LDL, HDL, etc.

Additionally there are different particle sizes of each of these.

So LDL cholesterol particles can be one of two main "patterns"….LDL-A and LDL-B.

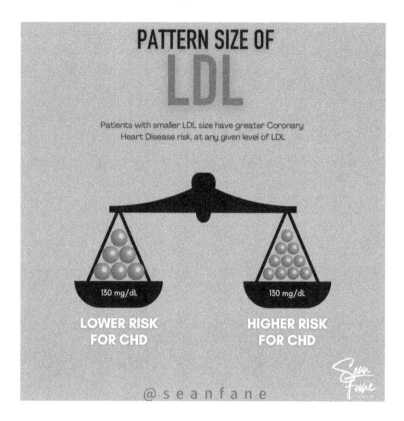

Our particle "pattern", like the quantity of your LDL and HDL, is genetic.......to start with.

LDL-A is a pattern of LDL distribution where more small, dense particles make-up the bulk of a person's LDL total.

These are ones that tend to remain lodged into artery walls after delivering their cholesterol "repair" cargo, and have more potential to become *oxidised* if we have created an inflammatory environment for them (like for example having an infection, oxidative damage from poor diet or hormonal imbalances).

LDL-B - is a pattern of LDL distribution where more large, benign particles make-up the bulk of a person's LDL total. These tend to resist oxidation and are less likely to lodge at the site of inflammation when they deliver their "repair" cargo.

If we have stress hormones rampaging through our blood, infections, pathogens or even have eaten inflammatory "foods" (like sugar and vegetable oil for example), this can create the environment that causes small LDL particles to oxidise.

This oxidisation is what damages our artery walls, and can instigate a "bodged"-repair job, which can become atherosclerosis.

And this is what causes a heart attack in most cases.

So the greater your pattern of LDL-A, the greater the risk that when the cholesterol is sent to heal any damage, it might lodge in your artery walls and oxidise, starting a cascade that could eventually lead to atherosclerosis.

The greater your pattern LDL-B, the less likely this is to happen.

What is interesting is *when we eat more saturated fat, and increase our overall cholesterol, we actually increase our LDL-B to a greater degree than LDL-A, and as such we improve our pattern profile and reduce our heart disease risk.*

I know what you're thinking….ditch the skimmed milk and pass me the cream!

That was the effect of increased cholesterol on LDL, but what about HDL?

Well again there is some good news here for those that consume more saturated fat.

HDL has a size issue too.

It is widely regarded as an important fact that HDL to LDL and HDL to Triglyceride ratios will predict heart disease risk.

The higher the HDL relative to these other measurements, the lower the ratio number, the lower the risk.

There is also a significant impact from the size of HDL particles as a study entitled ***Reduced HDL particle size as an additional feature of the atherogenic dyslipidemia***[8] from the ***Journal of Lipid Research*** confirms.

In technical jargon they say……

"Results of this study indicated that HDL particle size was a significant correlate of several features of an atherogenic dyslipidemic profile."

"Thus, men with large HDL particles had a more favourable plasma lipoprotein-lipid profile compared with those with smaller HDL particles. Furthermore, men with large HDL particles were also characterized by reduced overall adiposity and lower levels of visceral AT as well as reduced insulinemic-glycemic responses to an oral glucose load."

"In conclusion, small HDL particle size appears to represent another feature of the high TG-low HDL cholesterol dyslipidemia found in viscerally obese subjects characterized by hyperinsulinemia."

In layman's terms….what this means is smaller HDL signified poor metabolic function and increased risk of all the factors that lead to atherosclerosis.

So for both LDL and HDL, the most important thing is not to reduce them or remove them….*it is to optimise them, improve the ratio of HDL to LDL and increase the particle sizes of both of them.*

---

[8]   https://www.jlr.org/content/42/12/2007.short

Luckily, all of these objectives are achieved with one simple to remember dietary approach.

Eat more saturated fat, and eat less sugar!

INFLAMMATION

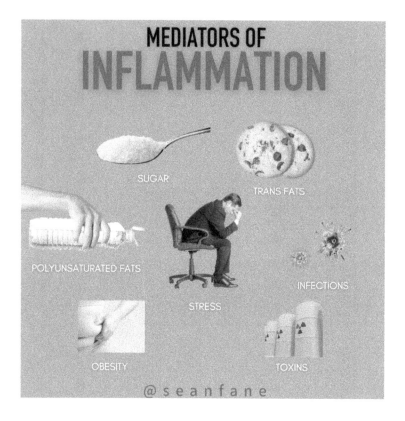

Inflammation is the first stage in the wound-healing process and can be recognised through heat, redness, pain, swelling, raised temperature and fever.

The function of inflammation is to neutralise and destroy any toxic agents at the site of an injury and restore tissue that has been damaged.

Inflammation is part of our bodies response to harmful stimuli, such as pathogens, damaged cells, or irritants, and can involve recruiting immune cells, blood vessels, and molecular mediators to help with the repair work.

If we didn't have any inflammation, then our wounds would never heal and we would never get over the flu or fight off bacterial infections, so inflammation is a good thing.

But like many things that are good for us in small doses, inflammation can be extremely damaging if it is allowed to continue for too long.

For example, when you make toast you expose bread to heat, until it gets nice and brown and crispy. Perfect! But leave the bread in the toaster too long you have a black lump of inedible charcoal.

And so it is with inflammation.

It is referred to as either acute inflammation (short periods of positive healing) or chronic inflammation (longer periods of damaging cell activity).

Acute inflammation is is achieved by the increased movement of plasma and things called leukocytes, from the blood into injured tissues to stimulate repair, and lasts for a few days.

So if you have a cut on your knee, for example, you will notice that over the first few days the area will become slightly swollen, warm and red as your body starts the process. This is inflammation, fending-off bacteria, sending in repair agents and altering blood-flow and white blood cell activity in the area.

Chronic inflammation, is a prolonged repair activity which leads to an alteration in the type of cells present, such as mononuclear cells, and this simultaneously destroys and heals tissue.

Chronic inflammation, therefore, becomes damaging, and can often continue for months and even years.

Infections and injuries trigger the body's immune response, and immune cells called macrophages produce free-radicals while fighting off invading germs.

This is a term you may have heard as oxidative stress.

Oxidation is a trigger for chronic inflammation.

You know something about oxidation already, as you see it when a freshly cut piece of apple turns brown.....almost like rusting, it is a chemical reaction occurring.

Overproduction of free radicals can cause oxidative damage to bio-molecules, (lipids, proteins, DNA), eventually leading to many chronic diseases such as atherosclerosis, cancer, diabetes, rheumatoid arthritis, cardiovascular diseases, strokes, etc.

So what causes oxidation and triggers inflammation?

Infections, food we eat, the air we breathe, the chemicals we are exposed to.....and the chemical reactions in our brains from stressors.

Even something as seemingly benign as gum disease[9] can be the trigger for an inflammatory response, that leads to heart disease.

It has been discovered that oxidative-inflammatory reactions even occur in subjects with anxiety, contributing to an alteration of survival responses and shorter life span.

In studies on mice[10], premature ageing and shorter life expectancy was the result of a poor response to stress and high levels of anxiety, triggering oxidative stress in their immune cells and tissues.

---

[9]   https://pubmed.ncbi.nlm.nih.gov/15699278/

[10]   https://pubmed.ncbi.nlm.nih.gov/24588831/

Researchers concluded that,

"This model supports the hypothesis that anxiety can be a situation of chronic oxidative stress and inflammation, especially in brain and immune cells, and this accelerates the rate of ageing."

Anti-oxidants are molecules that protect other molecules from oxidation.

Anti-oxidants are usually present in a variety of foods, and can be taken naturally, or in greater levels through supplementation.

A fundamental role for inflammation, has been established in mediating all of the stages of heart disease, from initiation through progression and, ultimately, the complications that lead to death (arrhythmia, atherosclerosis, clotting, arterial fibrillation, etc) .

Many heart attacks involve a chronic inflammatory response to damage in the artery walls, often triggered by oxidation.

Atherosclerosis is the process of artery wall thickening, in an attempt to heal damage, caused by inflammation.

Thrombosis occurs when blood clots block veins or arteries, which may be as a result of the atherosclerosis.

It has been highlighted in research that elevated markers of inflammation in blood tests accurately predict many acute coronary syndromes, independently of actual cardiac damage.

In other words, whether you currently look like you have heart disease or not, if your blood tests show that you have inflammation within your body, you are at high-risk for developing heart disease.

HS-CRP is such a marker that can be tested for, and demonstrates that inflammation is occurring in your body.

HS-CRP stands for High Sensitivity C-Reactive Protein and is often cited as a key indicator of the potential for heart disease risk if it remains high.

LP-PLA2 is another inflammatory marker that strongly predicts heart disease.

Chronic inflammation that is allowed to go un-checked for long periods of time can cause cellular damage, and can also create opportunities for bacteria and pathogens to penetrate the site of such damage, so it is important to make sure that inflammation, even from things that you may consider trivial, like gum disease, are not left to persist.

That is why, when you read a study or article with a dramatic headline such as **Gum Disease Can Increase Heart Disease Risk!** [11] they can often be more credible than they might, at first, seem.

Chronic inflammation anywhere in your body may become the catalyst for what eventually results in heart disease.

One of the things that you can do to reduce inflammation is to heal more quickly.

Now I know you are probably wondering how you might do that without X-Men-like powers, but it is often as simple as keeping your immune system working well, and maintaining good hygiene practices.

Gum disease is a great example, because many people allow gum disease to create chronic inflammation for a long time without really dealing with it, when a few simple steps can eradicate it quite quickly…such as;

---

[11]   https://www.bhf.org.uk/informationsupport/heart-matters-magazine/medical/oral-health

1. Eat less sugar (which impairs your immune system and feeds bacteria…a double whammy)

2. Brush your teeth twice a day

3. Floss regularly

4. If your gum disease persists, see a dental hygienist

Simple, right!?

Often some other forms of inflammation are a little less easy to spot, however, and you may not know that you have chronic inflammation occurring somewhere in your body.

So what are the tell-tale signs of chronic inflammation?

Here are a few things to look out for:

1. Body pain, arthralgia (joint pain), myalgia (muscle pain)

2. Chronic fatigue and insomnia (sleeplessness)

3. Depression, anxiety and mood disorders

4. Gastrointestinal complications like constipation, diarrhoea, and acid-reflux

5. Weight gain or weight loss

6. Frequent infections

Don't let issues like these become a part of your life.

Get these problems dealt-with and allow yourself time to recover from them, to ensure that you don't create a haven for chronic inflammation within your body which may inflict more serious health issues for your heart further down-the-line.

Another great strategy is to try to avoid many of the common causes of inflammation, so it doesn't occur in the first place.

In the ***Environmental Toxins***, ***Food*** and ***Lifestyle*** sections, later in this book, some of the key risk areas for inflammation will be highlighted.

One that we don't cover separately, I will mention here.

Fat cells are inflammatory, so anybody that is obese has a greater degree of inflammation by remaining in this state.

Ben Bikman describes in his book ***Why We Get Sick*** that;

"Fat tissues produce cytokines. These turn-on inflammatory processes and innocent fat cells become dangerous fat cells called ceramides."

Ceramides are known to impair a cells ability to use glucose, as fuel and stimulate something called insulin resistance.

Also in the ***Food*** section some very dangerous inflammatory substances will become apparent.

When doctors worry about your cholesterol, and in particular your LDL, and the particle size, it is because oxidised LDL can create an inflammatory process.

As you know by now, if you have damage to an artery wall cholesterol is sent to repair the damage in an LDL taxi.

If you have small particle sized LDL, and if that LDL is experiencing oxidation from some of the lifestyle factors, or bacteria or disease, then it can become lodged in your artery wall and trigger inflammation, which in turn creates the cascade of atherosclerosis (thickening of the arteries).

From this point on, the cascade can include problems such as; blood-clotting, plaque rupture, complete blockage, and more issues, any one of which can lead to a heart attack.

The solution is not to eradicate cholesterol or LDL, but to reduce the inflammation and improve your LDL particle size.

Over the course of the latter part of this book, we will discuss the various lifestyle and diet interventions that reduce inflammation, and create a positive hormone balance, and as a result, dramatically reduce your risk of heart disease.

ENVIRONMENTAL TOXINS

Nan's Chapter Summary: Environmental toxins contribute to heart disease by creating a "rusting" inside us known as oxidation.

Air pollution from car and factory fumes, wood burners, coal fires and mould, as well as lead, arsenic and cadmium can contribute to this problem.

Minimise your exposure to household air pollutants (and reduce carbon emissions) by removing all biomass heating systems and cooking systems in your home!

Minimise your exposure to ambient air pollution by living, working & socialising in a more rural setting if at all possible.

If you have mould in your home, make it a priority to get it treated or removed.

Avoid tobacco smoke and re-decorate old homes (carefully) with a focus on removing paintwork that may contain lead. Replace any old lead water pipes in older buildings.

Wash your rice and vegetables before cooking and be sure you know where your drinking water comes from.

Wash your vegetables and don't smoke!

Environmental exposures to toxins that can have a negative impact on your health can be a difficult challenge.

We take roughly 20,000 breaths per day.

If you live in the city for example, how can you avoid air pollution?

If you live in an old block of flats, is the water pumped to your apartment clean, or does it contain toxins, bacteria, heavy metals or pathogens that can trigger inflammation?

In low- and middle-income countries, where increased economic development and industrialisation is moving quickly, but maybe health and environmental standards are lower, there is a rising burden of cardiovascular disease as a consequence of greater exposure to environmental toxins.

But even in developed countries, increasing evidence suggests an association of exposure to ambient air pollution, household air pollution from biomass fuel, lead, arsenic, and cadmium with multiple cardiovascular disease outcomes including hypertension, coronary heart disease, stroke, and cardiovascular mortality.

Understanding the impact of environmental exposures on cardiovascular disease has the potential to yield greater insight into the full human cost of economic development, but economic development is unlikely to stop, so one must do what one can to mitigate against some of the most likely environmental toxins.

Some of the most harmful environmental toxins are through air pollution and exposure to cadmium, arsenic and lead.

A 2018 study[12] looked at the impact on CVD for the following 5 environmental exposures: air pollution, household air pollution, lead, arsenic, and cadmium.

Here is how they interpreted the impact of environmental toxins on heart disease:

Ambient Air pollution

Ambient air pollution affects cardiovascular health largely due to systemic inflammation from the incorporation of fine particles into the lungs and pulmonary system.

---

[12]   https://www.ncbi.nlm.nih.gov/pmc/articles/PMC5129872/

Exposure to ambient air pollution is associated with multiple measures of subclinical cardiovascular disease such as atherosclerosis including carotid-thickness and aortic atherosclerotic plaques. In other words narrowing the arteries of the brain and the heart.

Acute air pollution exposure has been associated with angina, stroke, acute myocardial infarction, heart failure hospitalisation, arrhythmias, cardiac arrest and cardiovascular mortality. So pretty much every different type of heart disease that there is.

Strategy - Minimise your exposure to ambient air pollution by living, working & socialising in a more rural setting if at all possible.

Household Air Pollution

Biomass fuels including wood, charcoal, dung and crop residue, which are burned in indoor and outdoor stoves for cooking and heating are implicated in heart disease.

Similar to fossil fuel combustion, biomass fuels produce gases and particles that are suspended in air. Exposure to the components of biomass fuel combustion has been studied in several contexts in relation to cardiovascular disease risk-factors and outcomes.

Household air pollution from biomass fuel use affects 3 billion people worldwide.

Acute exposure to wood smoke has been shown to cause arterial stiffness and decrease heart rate variability. Additionally, observational studies conducted in women in villages in eastern India observed increased pro-inflammatory cytokines, higher serum c-reactive protein, and higher reactive oxygen species generation in the women exposed to biomass fuel smoke.

The most common cardiovascular risk-factor associated with biomass fuel use is elevated blood pressure.

Strategy - Minimise your exposure to household air pollutants (and reduce carbon emissions) by removing all biomass heating systems and cooking systems in your home!

Household Mould

You now have an added incentive to get a bit of DIY completed and remove any mould that you have noticed around your house.

It has been known for a long time that mould is toxic, and that some people are particularly sensitive to household mould.

Common complaints to mould exposure include; nasal stuffiness, throat irritation, coughs, wheezing, eye irritation and skin irritation.

Some people have mould allergies, which may make reactions worse than others.

People with compromised immune systems or chronic lung illnesses, may suffer very serious lung infections when they are exposed to mould.

Mould is also an environmental toxin that can play a part in accelerating heart disease through its role as an inflammatory agent though.

In their blog relating to mould in the home, Environment.com state;

"Originally, toxic effects from mould were thought to be the result of exposure to the mycotoxins of some mould species, such as Stachybotrys chartarum. However, studies are suggesting that the so-called toxic effects are actually the result of chronic activation of the immune system, leading to chronic inflammation."

Dave Asprey also has some tips on how to eradicate the harmful effects of mould in his bulletproof.com website, where he explains;

"Mould toxins have been linked to damaging long-term effects including memory loss, insomnia, anxiety, depression, trouble concentrating, and even cancer and heart disease."

Strategy - If you have mould in your home, make it a priority to get it treated or removed.

Lead Exposure

Globally, an estimated 26 million people are at risk for lead toxicity. This results in 9 million disability-adjusted life-years lost.

Lead pipes and paint are common exposure mechanisms, and although reduced in common modern standards the prevalence of lead exposure has not decreased in low/middle income countries as much as many high-income countries.

Tobacco use is also a common mode of lead exposure.

Lead increases oxidative stress in cardiovascular tissues and endothelial cells (the cells of your artery walls). It is also associated with decreased nitric oxide (NO) availability, making it a vaso-constrictor (in other words it tightens your arteries). It also leads to the oxidation of LDL, increases the expression of adhesive molecules on monocytes and increases foam cell formation.

All of this means lead contributes quite heavily (excuse the pun) to tightening and damaging artery walls and then oxidising the LDL that goes to repair the damage.

This makes lead, pretty much, the perfect end-to-end heart-attack toxin.

Strategy - Avoid tobacco smoke and re-decorate old homes (carefully) with a focus on removing paintwork that may contain lead. Replace any old lead water pipes in old buildings.

Arsenic

I don't know about you, but I think of arsenic as some kind of industrial strength rat poison to which I am never exposed. I didn't even think there was an arsenic exposure issue for humans until researching for this book.

It turns out, arsenic is a naturally occurring metalloid and a contaminant of drinking water, soil, and food. It can be used in making glass and preserving wood.

It can be found in foods such as rice and vegetables, as well as some seafood.

Cigarettes are a factor too, according to a report from the California Air Resources Board and the Department of Health Services, smokers breathe in approximately 0.8 to 2.4 micrograms of inorganic arsenic per pack of 20 cigarettes.

Chronic arsenic exposure has been found in countries of all income levels.

In contrast to acute arsenic poisoning, chronic arsenic exposure can be more difficult to identify, but is ultimately association with multiple adverse health outcomes, including cardiovascular disease.

Arsenic typically enters the body through the gastrointestinal tract and is metabolised in the liver. Arsenic exposure is associated with increased inflammatory markers.

It damages the endothelial walls and elevates blood pressure, as well as increasing artery wall thickness which aggravates atherosclerosis.

*Strategy - **Wash your rice and vegetables before cooking and be sure you know where your drinking water comes from.***

Cadmium

An estimated 5 million people are chronically exposed to cadmium.

Similar to lead, cadmium exposure commonly occurs from tobacco smoking. Additionally, cadmium from mining, smelting, refining and industrial waste can also pollute air, water, and soil leading to the contamination of foods including leafy vegetables, fish, and shellfish.

Cadmium increases oxidative stress and has been shown to impair endothelial function.

Similar to other environmental exposures, cadmium exposure is associated with elevated blood pressure.

The evidence regarding the association between cadmium exposure and cardiovascular disease comes from high-income countries.

Cadmium exposure is associated with diseases of atherosclerosis including peripheral arterial disease, stroke, ischaemic heart disease, and acute coronary syndromes.

Again it is a significant environmental toxin contributing to heart disease.

Strategy - *Wash your vegetables and don't smoke!*

So here is a summary of some of the mechanisms by which environmental toxins can impact your heart health.

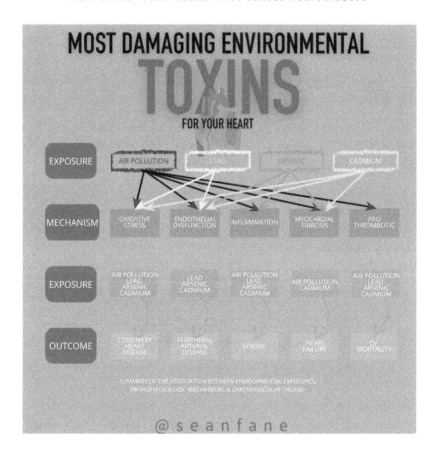

Increasing evidence suggests an association of exposure to ambient air pollution, household air pollution from biomass fuel, lead, arsenic, and cadmium with multiple cardiovascular disease outcomes including hypertension, coronary heart disease, stroke, and cardiovascular mortality.

Using some of the strategies here you can reduce the impact of these hidden toxins on your health.

FOOD

Nan's Chapter Summary: *The food that we eat can either harm us or nurture us.*

It is often very difficult to judge the harm that food does to us, as it occurs slowly over a long period of time, and we don't notice the negative effects until it is too late.

The foods that create the worst outcomes for our heart health are those that increase our production of a hormone called insulin, and also processed foods that contain negative ingredients and toxins that contribute to inflammation of our bodies.

Insulin is increased by eating foods that contain too much starch, or sugar.

We eat foods like this all the time, like pasta, bread, rice, potatoes, cereal, cakes, biscuits, fruit juice and carbonated drinks.

These foods create high blood sugar, which is dangerous, and can lead to type 2 diabetes, which can be fatal. Type 2 diabetes is a major factor in heart disease and a growing problem in general, and even though we may not be diabetic, many adults in the western world are on the road to becoming diabetic, or increasing their heart-disease risk by eating too many foods that raise blood sugar.

The other type of foods that damage our heart-health are processed foods containing things like seed oils, that we call vegetable oils.

These are oils like sunflower oil, canola oil, sesame oil, etc.

These oils are extracted from seeds using dangerous chemicals, and they are full of fats called 'omega 6', which are damaging to the body in high quantities.

We shouldn't really use these oils for cooking or in food, but instead use things like butter, coconut oil and olive oil instead.

Before we get into the nitty-gritty of food it might be helpful to start with a little mental re-adjustment to what food really is.

Food is just anything we consume from which we can derive the macro-nutrients and micro-nutrients we need to perform the chemical processes of functioning optimally.

Food is defined by Google as ***Any nutritious substance that people or animals eat or drink, or that plants absorb, in order to maintain life and growth.***

We need to bear this in-mind when going through this section of the book, because food is perhaps the single biggest element of "consumption" that we can control, and also has more power to heal or harm us every day than anything else.

Now not everything we put into our mouth is food.

For example, if we eat cardboard it will probably be relatively benign, because besides small quantities of glue it is pretty much paper, so eventually it will come out the other end (so to speak).

But it's not food because it provides no macronutrients, micronutrients or beneficial properties such as vitamins or minerals, and so we don't think of it as food. But if we eat it our bodies will process it in the same way that they processes all other substances we put in our mouths.

Our bodies will look for pathogens or toxins and try to neutralise them, look for nutrients to extract them, and discard the rest as waste.

If we eat enough cardboard consistently, it would be reasonable to assume that eventually we will suffer from health problems, because there are very few nutrients in cardboard and it does contain a few substances that are toxic.

Some health problems may arise from the chemical ingredients in cardboard, and some problems may be caused by the lack of nutrients we experience as a consequence of eating cardboard instead of real nutritious food. But if you eat it once, then no real problems will be visible immediately.

This was a strange example, I know, but it highlights that we think of substances with more toxins and less nutrients as non-food, like cardboard, and substances with more nutrients and less (or no) toxins as food.

So what is poison?

Basically it is something that falls into the non-food category. Something that in relatively small quantities will become damaging or fatal.

Poison is defined by Google as; ***A substance that is capable of causing the illness or death of a living organism when introduced or absorbed.***

In biochemistry, a poison is thought of as a substance, that causes damage to living tissues and has an injurious or fatal effect on the body, whether it is ingested, inhaled, or absorbed or injected through the skin.

In other words it becomes toxic.

Toxicity is the degree to which a chemical substance or a particular mixture of substances can damage an organism.

Toxicity can refer to the effect on a whole organism, such as an animal, bacterium, or plant, as well as the effect on a substructure of the organism, such as a cell or an organ such as the liver.

A central concept of toxicology is that the effects of a toxicant are ***dose-dependent*** so even water can be toxic when taken in too high a dose.

Toxicity is also species-specific, making cross-species analysis problematic, because, for example, something toxic to a dog like raisins or chocolate, may not be toxic to humans.

The things we call food......and anything else we consume, in the right quantities can become poisonous to us...and toxic.

Water for example is critical for life. If we are deprived of water, for long enough, we may die of de-hydration. We need water.

A little water is good, a lot is even better, but too much water and we can actually die of water toxicity.

Protein is critical for life. If we are deprived of protein for long enough we may suffer many terrible side effects before we finally succumb to organ failure. We need protein.

A little protein is good, a lot is even better, but too much protein in the blood (a very rare condition caused by some medical interventions) can cause pain, discomfort and fat storage. (You needn't worry about this, as it isn't related to how much you eat it is a rare genetic condition).

Fat in the diet is critical for life. If we are deprived of fat we can suffer heart problems, vitamin deficiencies (some important vitamins are fat soluble) mood changes, cognitive decline (mental impairment).

What if we have too much fat in the diet?

Well actually I can't find much real "legitimate" reference material for the negative health consequences of too much dietary fat.

If you Google "too much dietary fat", there are lots of articles, like this one in Medline Plus [13] called *Facts about saturated fats*, which states that;

"Your body needs healthy fats for energy and other functions". which is correct, but then it follows this up with *"But too*

_____

much saturated fat can cause cholesterol to build up in your arteries (blood vessels)." which is a completely untrue statement.

Eating saturated fat does NOT cause cholesterol to clog-up our arteries.

There is no scientific basis for this statement (which is why there is no reference material to back up the statement) but this is pretty much all you can find in most articles when trying to understand the real impact of too much dietary fat.

This kind of erroneous journalism is very common, and is partly due to the institutional beliefs around saturated fat that I covered earlier.

So where could one find examples of people that eat huge quantities of fat, so we can understand the recorded consequences of them doing so?

If eating fat was as dangerous as mainstream media believes, then there would presumably, be no people that fit this category. If there were, they would surely have succumbed to horribly blocked arteries, and they would lead the world in heart disease and early death.

Well the French eat a lot of fat.

About twice as much as most of the rest of Europe according to **The French Paradox**, but although they had the highest fat consumption in Europe (over the period measured for the analysis that lead to the moniker, along with the Swiss) they had about the lowest rates of heart disease.

Check-out The French Paradox[14] where it is noted **The existence of the French paradox has caused some researchers to**

---

speculate that the link between dietary consumption of satu-rated fats and coronary heart disease might not be as strong as had previously been imagined. This has resulted in a re-view of the earlier studies which had suggested this link.

Then of course there are Eskimo's....don't they live on seal blub-ber?

That is grade A saturated fat!

When researching to find what terrible medical fates must have be-fallen the Inuit Eskimo's (a tribe of Eskimo's for whom about 80% of their diet was from seal blubber and the rest oily fish) I didn't find much evidence of disease at all.

Look them up....here[15] where the *Inuit Paradox* is explained.

NB. It is only a paradox ....French or Inuit.....if one holds a misguided belief relative to the causes of heart dis-ease in the first place! Otherwise it is just logical.

Inuit diets have recently become more Westernised, their fats re-placed by processed foods and carbohydrates.....and unsurprisingly their incidence of heart disease and cancer have shot-up to almost Western society levels accordingly.

The price one pays for modernisation.

When something is a true food the quantities required to create harm may be huge, even beyond ones ability for consumption, and the benefits are obvious.

---

[15]   https://www.discovermagazine.com/health/the-inuit-paradox

Where things are highly toxic and poisonous, the damage is generally seen very quickly, and the quantities required to cause harm are very small.

Think of snake venom. Top of the list for poison!

So all of this brings us on to the stuff that we call "food" which actually isn't really designed to be eaten at all, and certainly not in the quantities we now consume.

Sugar

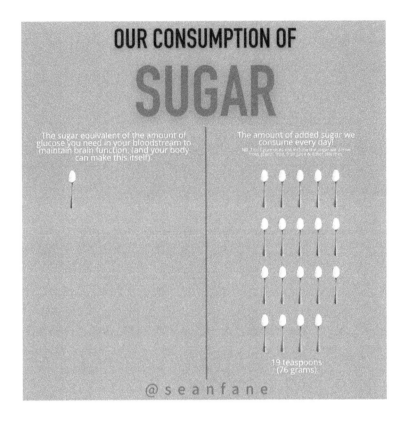

"Sugar is uniquely toxic, perhaps having prematurely killed more people than all wars combined." - Gary Taubes

Sugar isn't food!

Table sugar, the white granular substance we add to food and drinks, is a combination of two saccharides fructose and glucose (almost 50/50).

There is no nutritional value in sugar whatsoever.

It has no vitamins!

It has no minerals!

It has no amino acids!

It has not fats!

By definition, sugar isn't food.

Sugar is….by definition, poison!

It is similar to cardboard in nutritional quality….except that it has three negative elements that cardboard doesn't have.

1. It has calories…so it truly displaces real foods when we eat it, as we have a limit to how many calories we can reasonably consume.

2. It contains fructose… which demands our valuable resources and requires our liver to convert it into glucose (fructose itself cannot be utilised by the body) which stops the liver doing all the other things that it should be doing to keep you healthy (like filtering blood, producing cholesterol, etc).

3. It has a hormonal cost…..as our body fights to deal with an imbalance of excess glucose in the blood (which is extremely dangerous) we overproduce hormones like insulin and cortisol to facilitate removal of the glucose.

Excess blood glucose leads to death!

Our bodies fight hard to keep our blood glucose in balance, but when we put too much strain on this system, through constant excessive consumption of sugar and other blood glucose-raising "foods" we become, first insulin resistant, and later…when the pancreas and our cells are totally overwhelmed, we become type 2 diabetic…and then we either inject insulin forever or die.

Remember the definition of poison; *A substance that is capable of causing the illness or death of a living organism when introduced or absorbed.*

Whilst we sometimes get a short amount of pleasure from sugar at the time of eating it, it is also pretty damaging to our mental wellbeing, mood and cognitive function [16].

Chris Kresser MD states;

"Excessive sugar contributes to aggression, attention-deficit/hyperactivity disorder (ADHD), and bipolar disorder. This won't be a news flash to you, but believe it or not, the idea that sugar contributes to behavioural disorders is still controversial in the conventional medicine community. Hopefully, this [17] study (entitled Could excessive sugar intake contribute to aggressive behaviours, ADHD, bipolar disorder?) will help to shift that perception."

It is pretty tasty though…addictive even.

Gary Taubes writes;

"Sugar elicits the same responses in the nucleus accumbens (the brains reward centre) as do nicotine, cocaine, heroin and alcohol".

"Sugar stimulates the release of the same neurotransmitters, dopamine in particular, through which the actions that require the survival of the species (specifically eating and sex) are experienced as pleasurable in parts of the brain."

"Rats given sweetened water in experiments find it significantly more pleasurable than cocaine, even when they're addicted to cocaine in the first place. Offered the choice of a sweet solution or its daily cocaine fix and the rat will switch over to the sweet solution within two days."

In 1890, Robert Saundby a former president of the Edinburgh Royal medical Society, presented a series of lectures on diabetes to the Royal College of physicians in London in which he estimated that less than one in every 50,000 people died from diabetes.

"It is one of those rarer diseases." he said.

One Los Angeles physician, according to Saundby, reported in seven years practice he had;

"Not met with a single case."

In 1892, William Osler at John Hopkins Hospital in Baltimore reported that of the 35,000 patients treated at the hospital, only 10 had been diagnosed with diabetes.

In the next eight years 156 cases were diagnosed.

Mortality statistics for diabetes showed a nearly doubling between 1870 and 1890 and then more than doubling again by 1900.

In 2010 they were 73,000 *amputations* in the US alone through diabetes.

Those afflicted with diabetes will die at greatly increased rates from heart disease or stroke, from kidney disease and diabetic coma.

Type 2 diabetes is a disease entirely created by human diet and lifestyle.

Since Christopher Columbus first brought sugar to the New World on his second voyage in 1493, it has been exciting minds and fuelling bodies (although initially it was so expensive that it was never able to be consumed in large quantities).

In 1847 a Bostonian, Oliver Chase launched the modern 'candy' industry with his invention of a machine for producing candied lozenges in large quantities.

During a similar timeframe the Lindt brothers had worked-out how to solidify, and mass-produce, chocolate bars for distribution.

Welcome to the age of factory produced sweets!

The New York Times observed in 1884 by sweetening with sugar;

"We can give false palatable mess to even the most indigestibly rubbish."

By 1903, The New York Times had estimated the yearly candy industry to be worth $150m a year in the United States, up from nothing 25 years before.

In 1904 the ice cream cone was launched at the World's Fair in St Louis.

And of course Dr Pepper, Coca Cola and Pepsi were by then well on their way to global sales-reach, having been established in the 1880's.

By the 1920s sugar refineries we are producing as much sugar in a single day (millions of pounds) as would have taken refineries in the 1820s and entire decade to do.

The taste-buds of the day won the war against the poisonous effects of sugar during this time. British physician Willoughby Gardner wrote in the British Medical Journal in the early 1920's that sugar was;

"One of the most valuable articles in the diet, and yet is to be avoided like poison by those prone to obesity diabetes or gout."

In the mid 1930s the US Congress passed the ***Sugar Act***.

The Sugar Act effectively guaranteed producing and refining sugar in the United States would always be a profitable business.

The Sugar Act put limits on domestic production, set quoters and allowed for subsidies to be paid to sugar producers.

Shocking as it may sound to us now, the US Department of Agriculture suggested that sugar would seem to be a food *"especially adapted to children because of their great activity."*

In the 1930's the Sugar Institute placed regular advertisements in newspapers and magazines promoting sugar as a *health food*, a 1930s equivalent of probiotics.

Sugar Institute advertisements pitched sugar as a means to build-up the immune system and fight-off colds. (The opposite is true).

In 1943 the industry formed a new non-profit organisation the Sugar Research Foundation (SRF).

The focus of the SRF would be educating the public on the merits of sugar while simultaneously funding research that would *"secure all known facts about sugar and its effects on the human system."*

Among the many researchers that the sugar industry would begin supporting during the war years, two of them, Ancel Keys at the University of Minnesota and Fred Stare founder of the Department of nutrition at Harvard, would become lifelong friends of the industry.

Stare and Keys would play a critical role in the 1960's and 1970's defending the place of sugar in a healthy diet and arguing against the idea that it could be a cause of chronic disease. (These are the same chaps that perpetuated the myth that saturated fat caused heart disease!)

Between 1963 and 1969 the Sugar Association spent more than $665,000 on research designed to force the FDA to remove cyclamates (artificial sweeteners) from the GRAS list (a US list of foodstuffs Generally Recognised As Safe), ensuring that this non-caloric sweeteners could not displace their power.

Although entirely safe, they claimed cyclamates were dangerous after lab tests in rats, on the human equivalent of *550 cans of soda a day* for years, had seen some male rats develop bowel cancer.

Ironically, the equivalent consumption of soda containing sugar would have killed the rats from diabetes in a much, much shorter timeframe, than the few that developed cancer!

Despite the evidence (provided to remove cyclamates from the list) being demonstrated absurd many years ago, they succeeded in protecting sugar from a healthier alternative sweetener, and cyclamates were banned in foods in the US.

Sugars, like sucrose and high fructose corn syrup (and any of the other 60 or so names for sugar), are fundamental causes of diabetes. They have unique physiological, metabolic and endocrinological (hormonal) effects in the human body.

FRUIT AND BLOOD
GLUCOSE

An indication of how the fruit you consume can dramatically affect your blood glucose levels

TYPE OF FRUIT	GI	GL	SERVING	EFFECT RELATIVE TO TEASPOONS OF SUGAR
Banana	62	16	120g	
Grapes	59	11	120g	
Apple	39	6	120g	
Watermelon	80	5	120g	
Nectarines	43	4	120g	
Apricots	34	3	120g	
Strawberries	40	3.8	120g	

Source: It is the glycemic response to, not the carbohydrate content of food that matters in diabetes and obesity' The glycaemic index revisited, Journal of Insulin Resistance 2016

@ s e a n f a n e

AGE's (Advanced Glycation End-products) are sugar-damaged proteins.

In the last years AGE's have received particular attention.

They are formed in high amounts in diabetes but also in a physiological organism during ageing. They have been implicated in numerous diabetes and age-related diseases.

As we get older, excess free sugars in our blood cause damage quicker than our body can repair itself.

Sugar also attacks collagen[18], the structural protein that's responsible for elasticity and strength of skin and repairing dead skin cells. Thus, excess sugar consumption can leave us with premature wrinkles and an ageing complexion[19].

After consuming sugar, our immune system is depressed for a few hours, meaning we are more susceptible to catching a variety of illnesses while riding that sugar wave. Not great in the current COVID-19 environment.

In fact, we increase our risk of a fatal outcome from COVID-19 by 230% if our blood glucose remains chronically high.

Ketogenic diets are far more beneficial in resolving high blood sugar than low-fat diets, as demonstrated in the meta-analysis titled ***Impact of a Ketogenic Diet on Metabolic Parameters in Patients with Obesity.***[20]

"Our study findings confirmed that ketogenic diets were more effective in improving metabolic parameters associated with glycemic, weight, and lipid controls in patients with overweight or obesity, especially those with pre-existing diabetes, as compared to low-fat diets."

Sugars create a chemical reaction with proteins, and interestingly fructose is 10 times more reactive, and more dangerous than glucose.

---

18   https://observer.com/2018/02/sugar-is-wreaking-havoc-on-your-hormonal-health/

19   https://www.ncbi.nlm.nih.gov/pmc/articles/PMC3583887/

20   https://pubmed.ncbi.nlm.nih.gov/32640608/

Since the 1970s we have been using increasingly more refined fructose (from high-fructose corn syrup amongst other things) in processed foods.

Its sweetness, and ability to suppress ghrelin (the hormone that tells you, you're "full") results in excessive food consumption[21].

It impairs our lipid circulation is contributes to obesity, and its associated with many health problems[22].

As Gary Taubes puts it in *The Case Against Sugar*

"The metabolism of fructose in the liver is "unfettered" by the cellular controls that would work to prevent its conversion to fat. This results in increased production of triglycerides and thus the abnormally elevated triglyceride levels that were observed in many research subjects when they eat sugar rich diet."

He continues, when describing the studies on fructose;

"Feed animals enough pure fructose and their livers convert much of it into fat (the saturated fat palmitic acid to be precise which is the one that supposedly gives us heart disease) when we eat it."

"Feed animals enough fructose for long enough and this fat accumulates in the liver causing the kind of fatty liver seen in obese children and adults the fat accumulation which accompanies insulin resistance."

It has been known since the 1960's that insulin resistance, which leads to type 2 diabetes, can be managed through reducing our bodies

---

21   https://pubmed.ncbi.nlm.nih.gov/18627777/

22   https://www.ncbi.nlm.nih.gov/pmc/articles/PMC3258689/

constant battle with high blood glucose caused by the glycemic roller-coaster that we put ourselves through with the massive over consumption of simple carbohydrates and sugar.

We "micro-dose" on a sweet-tasting poison that slowly kills us, and because the symptoms aren't visible until 20 or 30 years of abuse, we ignore it as a problem, and even "treat" ourselves and our children with more of it as a reward for good behaviour or an achievement.

3.5 million people in the UK have diabetes, and it is estimated that a further 549,000 people have it but are, as yet, undiagnosed [23].

The analogy of boiling a frog comes to mind. If you place a frog in boiling water, it will jump straight out!

If you place a frog in cold water, and slowly heat it on a stove, the frog will stay in the water until it boils to death.

We are the same with our diets and lifestyles when it comes to sugar.

Because we can't see the inevitable, horrendous consequences of eating a little sugar, we brush aside the thought of correcting bad food choices, and allow days, weeks, months and years of compound bad choices result in "an unexpected heart attack" or "type 2 diabetes".

Worse still, insulin resistance can become a genetic characteristic that is passed-down through generations, and it is shown that diabetic and pre-diabetic parents can pass poor glucose metabolism to their children to some extent, making this problem the biggest and fastest-growing health pandemic of all time.

John Yudkin wrote in 1963 of the situation in England;

---

[23]   https://www.diabetes.co.uk/diabetes-prevalence.html

"We now eat in two weeks the amount of sugar our ancestors of 200 years ago ate in a whole year. Sugar provides about 20% of our total intake of calories and nearly half of our carbohydrate."

There is a pillar of nutritional "wisdom" which is far more fundamental, and ultimately has far more influence on how the science has developed and it still dominates thinking on the sugar issue.

As such it has also done far more damage.

To the sugar injury industry, it has been the gift that keeps on giving, the ultimate defence against all arguments and evidence that sugar is uniquely toxic.

This is the misguided idea that we get obese or overweight because we "take-in" more calories than we expend.

By this thinking researchers and public health authorities think of obesity as an order of energy balance, a concept that has become so ingrained in conventional thinking, so widespread, that arguments to the country have typically been treated I was quackery if not a wilful disavowal of the laws of physics.

According to this flawed and overly simplistic logic of energy balance, of *calories-in* versus *calories-out*, the only meaningful way in which foods we consume have an impact on our body weight, and body fat is through their energy content.

We grow fatter because we eat too much (we consume more calories than we expend).

This simple explanation was, and still is, considered by many, all that is necessary to explain obesity and its prevalence in populations.

This thinking renders effectively irrelevant, the radically different impact that different macronutrients of foods have on metabolism, and on the hormones and enzymes that regulate our bodies, whether they burn fuel, are used to rebuild tissues and organs or are stored as fat.

With this energy balance logic, the close association between obesity diabetes and heart disease implies no profound revelations to be gleaned about underlying hormonal or metabolic disturbances.

Rather that obesity is driven, and diabetes and heart disease are exacerbated by some combination of gluttony and sloth.

Despite copious reasons to question this logic, and an entire European School of clinical research that came to consider it nonsensical, medical and nutrition "authorities" have tended to see it as the gospel truth.

They feel that obesity is caused by this caloric imbalance and diabetes is largely a penalty for obesity.

By the 1960s the phrase "a calorie is a calorie" had become the mantra of the nutrition establishment and it was invoked to make this argument, and it still is. Every fitness model or "personal trainer" will shout it from their Instagram feed.

In the 1920's and 1930's scientists Bergman and Bauer explored fat accumulation and its causes.

Their observations about obesity showed that caloric balance and a perverted appetite offered *"no meaningful explanation"* for fat accumulation.

In a series of articles Bauer argued that obesity was clearly the end result of dysregulation of the biological factors that normally work to keep fat accumulation in-check.

The first models in the 1930s identified that Bauer and Bergmans hormonal regulatory view on obesity was, in fact, correct.

Experiments at the time showed them that gluttony was not the cause of fat accumulation, but that hormones regulated energy expenditure and fat storage.

In the 1960's Rosalyn Yalow and Solomon Berson invented a technology to measure hormones in the blood. Yalow went on to win the Nobel Prize for the discovery.

This led to the discovery that nearly all hormones can mobilise fat (from fat cells) for energy.

Despite this, many believe that calories consumed or "burned" are what matters most for fat-loss.

Despite there being no reliable way to calculate a person's metabolic rate accurately, or the fact that up to 25% of the calories in protein are used converting it to energy, or the fact that calorie trackers can be "out" by more than 50%, an industry has developed of "nutritionists" and personal trainers that will assert that weighing food, and tracking calories-in v calories-out, is a sensible approach to weight loss.

This is a vanity, that in some ways mirrors its proponents personalities, and does not lead to good health outcomes. It will very often lead to clients of these health experts frustrated, hungry, nutritionally lacking and no better-off!

Eating whatever we want to eat (just in low enough quantities) but still being healthy and slim is a great sales message, and one we all want to hear, but unfortunately life doesn't work like that.

In order to obtain sufficient nutrients and protein and fats, we should not and cannot spend our lives in a constant "calorie deficit", let alone take-up some of the few calories we are "allowed" with a chocolate bar with zero nutrients "guilt-free".

Ask your PT or nutritionist to do this calculation for you.

Add up your supposed calorie allowance for a given day.

Then deduct the "250 calorie deficit" they will set, so you can lose weight.

Now take the balance and try to create a meal plan containing your RDA (even though RDA's for some vitamins are very low) for proteins, fat, carbohydrates and all the vitamins and minerals needed for good health.

Good Luck!

Insulin resistance, which leads to type 2 diabetes, is growing at an alarming rate!

There *is* something that can be done to reduce your propensity to insulin resistance and the onset of type 2 diabetes, or any of the other chronic diseases that are amplified or manifested from it, such as all heart disease and many cancers.

Reduce your insulin production by reducing your consumption of sugar and starches.

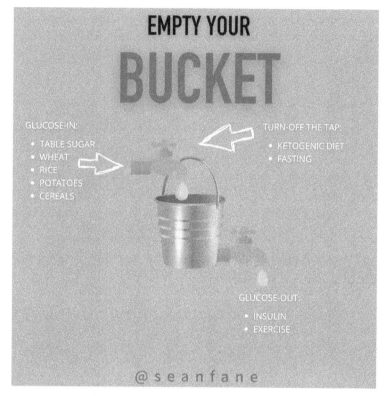

Let me summarise with a couple of studies:

In a study published in 2014 in JAMA Internal Medicine, Dr. Hu and his colleagues found an association between a high-sugar diet and a greater risk of dying from heart disease[24].

"Consuming too much added sugar can raise blood pressure and increase chronic inflammation, both of which are pathological pathways to heart disease."

---

24 https://www.health.harvard.edu/heart-health/the-sweet-danger-of-sugar

"The effects of added sugar intake — higher blood pressure, inflammation, weight gain, diabetes, and fatty liver disease — are all linked to an increased risk for heart attack and stroke."

Over the course of this 15-year study[25], people who got 17% to 21% of their calories from added sugar had a 38% higher risk of dying from cardiovascular disease compared with those who consumed 8% of their calories as added sugar.

Here are 5 tips to get you on the right path to reverse insulin resistance without the need for any drugs:

1. ***Don't have sugar in tea or coffee.*** It takes about 2 weeks to wean yourself off sugar in drinks, and when you do tea will taste just as good to you as it did before. If you have 3 or 4 cups of tea a day that is a lot of extra sugar avoided! It is thought that we add 19 teaspoons of sugar to our diets every day, and just dropping two teaspoons from 4 cups of tea a day may halve that. This might be the difference between a life without metabolic issues, or an eventual decline into insulin resistance and eventually diabetes, and all of the chronic terminal illnesses that follow. Is it really worth it!?

2. ***Find a new treat.*** When you want to reward yourself, do it with something that doesn't contain sugar. It is all too common for us to self-sabotage by treating! Hit the gym, then you deserve a chocolate bar as a treat! Cycle to the shops, come back

---

25

https://jamanetwork.com/journals/jamainternalmedicine/fullarticle/1819573

and have a few extra biscuits with your cuppa. Treats that elevate blood glucose will elevate insulin, reduce fat loss, increase appetite and work against your health. Have treats ready that aren't food-based, or if they are are, just not sugar-based….maybe create some healthy ketogenic treats like these almond protein balls [26] or these keto protein bars [27].

3. ***Skip breakfast!*** Forget what your mother told you! Breakfasts aren't the most important meal of the day, but they are the most damaging. They shorten the positive effects of the "fast" you have received whilst asleep, and if started with glucose will set you up for a roller-coaster ride of insulin and glucose interaction. Extending the time until the "break" in breakfast is shown to be a great way to massively improve your insulin sensitivity. Make lunch your first meal of the day and watch how your energy increases and your hunger subsides (great indicators that you are fixing your metabolism).

4. ***Skip puddings!*** It has been demonstrated that a sugar "fix" before bed can lead to poor quality sleep and a craving for more sugar in the morning. Whilst carbs do make you sleepy (especially if you don't have many throughout the day) like alcohol they can send you off to sleep initially, but will often interrupt sleep patterns and prevent deep sleep, leaving you groggy and tired. Wake-up without the sugar cravings and rumbly stomach, by skipping sugar before bed, and prevent the roller-coaster of cravings before it even starts.

---

[26] https://ketodietapp.com/Blog/lchf/healthy-keto-almond-protein-balls

[27] https://chocolatecoveredkatie.com/keto-protein-bars/

5. ***Empty your bucket!*** Think of your body as a bucket full of glucose...when it is being used through exercise (the bucket is being emptied), you are well, but when it is floating around your bloodstream (a full bucket) it is extremely damaging to you. Keep active, utilise any excess blood-sugar through exercise, and improve your insulin sensitivity. Make sure you get out walking, playing tennis or being generally physically active throughout the day to keep emptying your bucket. Short, intense resistance training or HIIT are particularly effective at ***emptying the bucket.***

In an ideal world, you would get the message and remove sugar entirely from your diet.

In the real world, be extremely conscious of the amount of excess sugar you are consuming, and also be aware that it is added to EVERY-THING!

If you already have heart disease, removing sugar from your diet would be pretty high, if not at the top, of my list of the first things you should do.

Carbohydrates

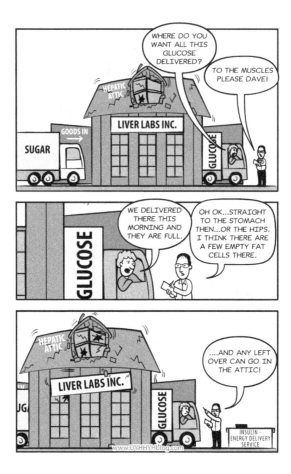

Carbohydrates are "foods" that we **can** use for energy.

There is a general perception that we **need** carbohydrates for energy. This is entirely untrue!

We are advised to eat carbohydrates to fuel our workouts, and provide us energy throughout the day.

They are considered one of the three essential macro-nutrients, along with proteins and fats, and are always mentioned as such in government nutritional guidelines.

In fact, ever since the **Food Guide Pyramid** was introduced by the United States Department of Agriculture in 1992, with a stated aim;

"to prevent obesity, improper nutrition and chronic diseases". (and was replaced by **My Plate** in 2011) the Western world has been advised to consume most of its dietary calories from grains, starches, wheat, rice, bread, etc. and pretty much avoid fat…certainly saturated fat.

Since then we have all done a great job of reducing our saturated fat intake, and indeed these calories have been replaced in our diets by starches such as pasta, cereals, bread, potatoes and rice.

Below is a picture of the Food Guid Pyramid from 1992, from which point, no doubt, it was expected that the adoption of these health guidelines would start to show a great improvement in the metabolic health of Americans (and the rest of us that followed their guidelines), as they became more educated on the healthiest foods to consume.

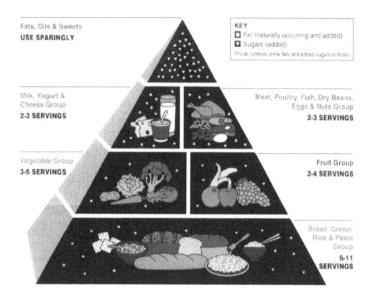

And here are the statistics for new cases of diabetes in adults between 1980 and 2015 in the United States.

CDC DIABETES STATISTICS

AS AMERICANS ARE ENCOURAGED TO EAT MORE GRAINS, DIABETES INCREASES

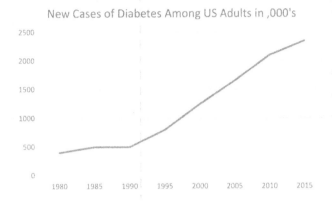

Introduction of The Food Guide Pyramid

New Cases of Diabetes Among US Adults in ,000's

Source: http://www.cdc.gov/diabetes/statistics/incidence

So in exactly the timeframe that we made the dietary changes that were designed to improve our metabolic health, we accelerated the epidemic of diabetes!

This shows correlation, not causation, but even if we didn't already have all of the science to back-up the relationship between high carbohydrate diets, elevated insulin and conditions like diabetes, it should be enough to make you question the conclusions that a diet rich in carbohydrates is healthy.

The fact that the food pyramid was not based on nutritional science or data, seems to have been overlooked, and is now resigned to history…..but that's another story. *NB (Read Nina Teicholz book The Big Fat Surprise for more on this…it is fascinating and a little frightening)!*

101

This is the presumed wisdom from the general population.

Running a marathon? Then we need to "carb-load" by eating our bodyweight in pasta the night before.

Going to the gym? Then we need a pre-workout shake with carbs in it to make sure we have enough energy to train hard!

We make a virtue of feeding our children fruit, pasta, rice, vegetables (basically a TONNE of carbohydrates) so they have the energy to play during the day….because we believe these things are healthy. Grains, starchy vegetables, fruit… are all natural… grown in soil, so they must be healthy..right? But do children need this type of food for energy?

One could write a whole book on this subject alone, but this is a heart disease book, so I won't go into too much detail….but the basic facts are these.

Whilst we need fats to enable us to thrive and survive, and we need amino acids from protein to enable us to thrive and survive, there is no requirement for carbohydrates to enable us to thrive….or to survive…..

…..or to run a marathon….

….or to train at the gym….

….or to walk to the tube…..

….or to fuel your children's growth or energy demands.

For the same reason that sugar is terrible for blood glucose levels, so are carbohydrates. They are made from glucose after all.

In fact, some carbohydrates elevate blood glucose (referred to sometimes as blood sugar) faster and higher than actual sugar.

FOOD AND BLOOD
GLUCOSE

An indication of how some foods we consume can dramatically affect our blood glucose levels

FOOD	GI	SERVING	EFFECT RELATIVE TO TEASPOONS OF SUGAR
Basmati Rice	69	150g	
Potato	96	150g	
Spaghetti	39	180g	
Wholemeal Bread	74	30g	
Broccoli	15	80g	Other foods in the very low range would include nutrient-dense foods such as oily fish, beef, cheese, mushrooms
Eggs	0	60g	

Source: It is the glycemic response to, not the carbohydrate content of food that matters in diabetes and obesity. The glycemic index revisited. Journal of Insulin Resistance 2016

@ s e a n f a n e

Half of sugar (table sugar) is fructose, which needs to travel to the liver to be converted into glucose before it can go into the bloodstream, so there is a small delay in it reaching the blood.

The sugars in carbohydrates are pretty much all glucose, so travel straight from the stomach to the blood.

For this reason, a slice of bread may have a faster and greater negative effect on your blood glucose than a bar of chocolate.

Measuring the effect of food on your blood glucose is performed through two measurements, glycemic load and glycemic index.

The glycemic index (GI) assigns a numeric score to a food based on how quickly it makes your blood sugar rise.

Foods are ranked on a scale of 0 to 100, with pure glucose given a value of 100.

The lower a food's glycemic index score, the *slower* blood sugar rises after eating that food.

The higher a food's glycemic index score, the *faster* blood sugar rises after eating that food.

What it doesn't tell you is how high your blood sugar could go when you actually eat the food. That is measured by the glycemic load.

Glycemic load (GL) estimates the impact of carbohydrate intake while taking into account the amount of carbohydrates that are eaten in a serving.

For instance, watermelon has a high GI, but a typical serving of watermelon does not contain many carbohydrates, it contains more fibre and water, so the glycemic load of eating it is relatively low.

Whereas glycemic index is defined for each type of food, glycemic load can be calculated for any size serving of a food, an entire meal, or an entire day's meals.

The glycemic load of a 100g serving of food can be calculated as its carbohydrate content measured in grams (g), multiplied by the food's GI, and divided by 100.

For example, watermelon has a GI of 72.

A 100 g serving of watermelon has 5g of available carbohydrates (it contains a lot of water), making the calculation $(5 \times 72)/100 = 3.6$, so the GL is rounded up to 4.

A food with a GI of 90 and 8g of available carbohydrates has a GL of 7.2 ($8 \times 90/100 = 7.2$), while a food with a GI of just 6 and with 120g of carbohydrate also has a GL of 7.2 ($120 \times 6/100=7.2$).

Calculating the GI or GL of a food is not something that I would recommend you do (I want to free you of this type of food and nutrient micro-management) but it is useful to know that all carbohydrates do not affect your body in the same way.

It is handy in general, however, to know which foods have a high GL, and try to minimise them, as they create the most challenges with insulin management, and provide the most opportunity for metabolic issues.

In general, think of carbohydrates in the same way that you think of sugar.

Less work for the liver, but more work for your pancreas, and creating elevated blood glucose, which elevates insulin, which is OK periodically, but not good thing if it is a constant state!

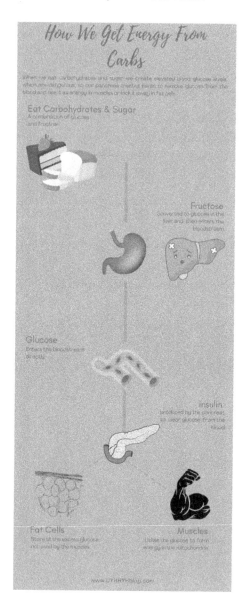

The picture above describes the effect of eating carbohydrates and sugar.

Once in the stomach all the glucose is delivered directly into our bloodstream, triggering our pancreas to secrete insulin. Insulin shuttles the glucose into muscles if they have storage space, or if they are active and require more energy. If the muscles are full and have enough glucose to operate, any excess glucose is stored in fat cells.

The fructose element of the sugar is sent to our poor, overworked liver, to convert to glucose, which has three potential destinations...our muscles...but again if they have sufficient, then the remaining glucose is stored in fat cells or in our liver will also store some.

When this system is over-worked and insulin resistance starts to take effect the liver becomes a store for fats and an over-accumulation of stored glucose in the liver, and the creation of fat cells in the liver can be referred to as "fatty liver" or Non-Alcoholic Fatty Liver Disease (NAFLD).

Here are some comments from one of the earlier mentioned studies *Food consumption and the actual statistics of cardiovascular diseases:* [28]

"The results of our study show that high-glycaemic carbohydrates or a high overall proportion of carbohydrates in the diet are the key ecological correlates of CVD risk."

"These findings strikingly contradict the traditional 'saturated fat hypothesis', but in reality, they are compatible with the evidence accumulated from observational studies that points to both high glycaemic index and high glycaemic load as important triggers of CVD."

---

[28]   https://www.ncbi.nlm.nih.gov/pmc/articles/PMC5040825/

Now, whilst it is logical to think of carbohydrates as sugar, as I tend to do, there will be a number of you that might wish to defend the consumption of certain types of carbohydrates.

We are, after all, bombarded by the advice to eat "healthy wholegrains" and fibre-rich diets and a diverse selection of fruit and vegetables.

There is a bit of a trade-off with carbohydrates, because unlike sugar they can contain positive nutrients and phytochemicals in varying degrees, along with water and fibre.

This is where judgment and a little knowledge goes a long way.

For example, carbohydrates can be broken down into a number of types for food; grains, starches, fruits, sugars, etc.

So you should understand that there is a difference between eating 100g of broccoli vs 100g of bread?

Both would be considered carbohydrates.

One is a natural, fibrous, low GL vegetable containing protein, iron, potassium, calcium, selenium and magnesium as well as the vitamins A, C, E, K and a good array of B vitamins including folic acid. (Broccoli).

The other is a processed food with a monstrous glycemic load, based on a genetically modified grain with limited nutrients and actually contains anti nutrients like phytic acid which prevent the absorption of vitamins and minerals. (Bread).

"Greater consumption of phytic acid has resulted from increased consumption of high fibre foods. If the consumer is eating a marginal diet in essential minerals, the phytic acid may lead to a nutritional deficiency (Lehrfeld, 1994)."

So the broccoli is great for health and the bread is a disaster for health. (And don't think for a second it makes a massive difference whether the bread is wholegrain or not....it really doesn't).

So herein lies the carbohydrate dilemma.

They aren't necessary for good health or energy, but some provide nutritional benefits (broccoli) and others are significant players in the development of insulin resistance and inflammation, and therefore, chronic diseases such as heart disease, diabetes, auto-immune disorders and most cancers (bread).

So what you need to learn is which ones to ditch (or limit)!

And in a nutshell it is these:

Potatoes, rice, pasta, cereals, beans, corn, wheat.

Maybe you already knew these carbohydrates were high starch, which means high sugar.

To those that claim that brown rice is better than white rice, and wholegrain bread is better than white bread, well, there is a point at which you need to understand that this is merely the difference between monumentally crappy outcomes and just crappy outcomes. The fact is both are high glycemic foods in the first place, and both stimulate insulin.

Even meta-analyses[29] that show a slight improvement from substituting one crappy genetically modified starch with a slightly less damaging variant based on colour or fibre content, don't change the basic metabolic damage caused by both.

"Inverse associations between several specific types of whole grains and type 2 diabetes warrant further investigations."

---

[29]   https://pubmed.ncbi.nlm.nih.gov/24158434/

A randomised controlled trial called ***Effect of Brown Rice, White Rice, and Brown Rice with Legumes on Blood Glucose and Insulin Responses in Overweight Asian Indians:***[30] sought to establish the differences in blood glucose effects from feeding white rice or brown rice to 15 overweight Asian Indians.

The change in glucose concentration was calculated on each test day for 5 days and averaged.

The results showed that;

*"**Average blood glucose** was was **19.8% lower in the brown rice group than in the white rice group.**"*

Marginally less crappy than the very high white rice score!

If you absolutely insist on eating rice, then it's is a slight improvement on a terrible food choice.

Definitely NOT a reason to make brown rice a staple food source.

White rice has a glycemic index of 65 and 29g of carbs per 100g, so the glycemic load of white rice is 18.85.

Brown rice has a glycemic index of 55 and 24g of carbs per 100g, so the glycemic load of brown rice is 13.2.

Ever tried making cauliflower rice? It is delicious and has a glycemic load of 10.

Ever tried courgetti-spaghetti, where you get spirals of courgette and use it instead of pasta or rice? Delicious and …wait for it.

Courgette has a glycemic index of 15 and 2g of carbs per 100g, so the glycemic load of courgette is a whopping *0.3.*

---

[30]   https://www.ncbi.nlm.nih.gov/pmc/articles/PMC3996977/

You can choose any of these as the base for a tasty beef or chicken or prawn curry.

You choice will be either terrible, a bit better, pretty good, or off-the-scale excellent!

The point is that if you want to protect yourself from the chronic adverse effects of insulin resistance there is an obvious choice.

Reduce or eliminate sugars and starchy foods from your diet.

Vegetable Oils

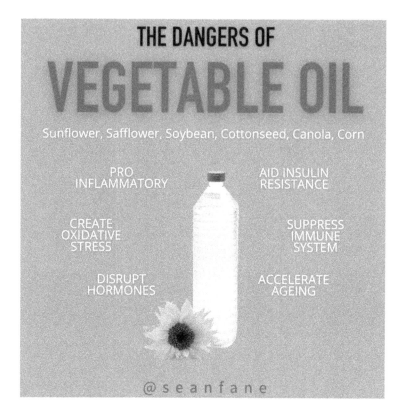

THE DANGERS OF
VEGETABLE OIL
Sunflower, Safflower, Soybean, Cottonseed, Canola, Corn

PRO
INFLAMMATORY

AID INSULIN
RESISTANCE

CREATE
OXIDATIVE
STRESS

SUPPRESS
IMMUNE
SYSTEM

DISRUPT
HORMONES

ACCELERATE
AGEING

@ s e a n f a n e

Vegetable oils are pretty much the last thing you should be putting into your body.

Aside from the obvious white and granular elephant in the room of course.

50 years ago paint and varnishes were made of soy, safflower and linseed oils, but then chemists learned how to make paint from petroleum, which was cheaper, which meant the vegetable oil industry had a lot of crops but without customers.

After initially giving the oils to farmers, to fatten livestock with less food, some smart-alec decided that maybe seed oils could be palmed-off as a healthy alternative to, the much vilified, butter.

Despite often being pitched as "heart-healthy" vegetable oils are anything but healthy.

Just to be clear, by vegetable oils I (and everybody else that refers to this strange group of oils as "vegetable" oils) am referring to a collection of oils extracted from a strange variety of non-food plants, for our consumption and for cooking. Let's call them seed oils, as many of them are derived from seeds.

Like sugar, they seem to have found their way into every piece of processed food imaginable, either to improve texture, preservation, taste or to bind foods together.

Try to find a processed food, treat, cake, health bar, sauce without sugar and vegetable/seed oil in the ingredients list.

According to Chris Knobbe MD, on *The Fat Emperor podcast 82* [31]

"Vegetable oils are indeed, bottled poison!"

"I say that because they are pro-inflammatory, pro-oxidative, toxic and nutrient deficient." he continued.

"Westernised diets can be defined as refined white flour, refined added sugar, polyunsaturated vegetable oils and trans fats, and in my opinion these four things make up man-made, nutrient-deficient, toxic food and are the drivers of all modern chronic disease."

---

[31]   https://thefatemperor.com/ep82-chris-knobbe-md-the-scientific-truth-behind-vegetable-oils-are-they-like-poison/

So a brief history of heart disease, and an uncanny alliance to the historic development of vegetable oil consumption.

John Hunter, a brilliant English physician of the eighteenth century, was probably the first in Western medicine to paint the clinical picture of chest pain, followed by a sudden death, which was termed angina pectoris.

Noting that his own symptoms of angina were aggravated by anger, he complained that his life was *"in the hands of any rascal who chose to annoy or tease him."*

Somewhat ironically, he proved his point by dying abruptly, after an argument with a fellow member the board at St. George's Hospital.

Myocardial infarction, a classic heart attack characterised by prolonged chest pressure or pain, followed by collapse with rapid death was put forward in the early part of the twentieth century.

In the 19th Century, *there were only two cases of myocardial infarction recorded*....one was in Switzerland in 1859.

Sir William Osler, one of the four founders of the John Hopkins Hospital, (a general practice hospital in Baltimore, Maryland) published a paper in 1897. Going back through his historical data from the previous 21 years of his hospital statistics, he had not experienced any sufferers of a heart attack and only 6 cases of angina.

13 years later in 1910, Osler presented at a medical conference in London, where he stated that an additional 208 cases of angina had been evidenced from 1897 to 1910, but he had still not recorded a single case of a heart-attack.

NB. (The earliest clinico-pathological report of CHD was in 1859, an anecdotal case report of myocardial infarction (MI) presented to the Swedish Medical Society.)

In 1912 James Herrick published the first case of a heart attack in the USA.

By the 1930's, 25 years later, heart attacks had become the leading cause of death in the United States.

America went from zero heart-disease to the first recorded myocardial infarction in 1912, to it accounting for 1 in 3 deaths in 2010.

Quite a leap, I am sure you will agree.

In the UK from 1900-1910 there were zero per 100,000 heart disease deaths, before the first cases arrived.

Between 1921 and 1927 coronary artery disease deaths doubled in the UK.

Between 1927 to 1929 they doubled again.

Between 1929 to 1933 they doubled again.

Between 1933 to 1939 they doubled again.

Between 1939 to 1948 they doubled again.

Between 1948 to 1956 they doubled again.

By 1970 550 people per 100,000 died in the UK from heart disease…up from zero 60 years before.

Coronary heart disease is currently responsible for around 63,000 deaths in the UK each year, an average of 170 people each day, or one death around every eight minutes.

In the UK, one in eight men and one in 13 women will die from coronary heart disease.

Coronary heart disease kills more than twice as many women in the UK as breast cancer.

So what happened between the latter part of the 19th Century to the early part of the 20th century to create this phenomena of chronic terminal illness?

Well there was the massive rise in consumption of sugar for sure.

But was there anything else?

Well, seed oils went from being completely unknown in 1910 to accounting for roughly 10% of the calories consumed by Americans today according to Knobbe.

These seed oils do lower cholesterol in the body, and because of this fact the American Heart Association has recommended their consumption since the 1960's.

As you are now aware of how misguided that advice has been, you will start to understand the terrible advice we have been asked to follow by organisations such as the AHA.

They recommend that Americans derive 5% to 10% of their calories from polyunsaturated oils, which is, I believe, incredibly damaging health advice.

This is a graph, demonstrating the uncanny parallels of heart disease deaths with relative consumption of vegetable oil and butter over the last century.

VEGETABLE OIL & HEART DISEASE

VEGETABLE OIL CONSUMPTION VERSUS HEART DISEASE DEATHS IN THE USA

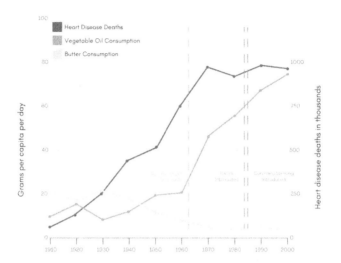

Source: The Displacing Foods of Modern Commerce: Are the Primary and Proximate
Cause of Age-Related Macular Degeneration A Unifying Singular Hypothesis

We swapped butter for margarine, seed oil consumption increased, butter consumption declined, and deaths from heart disease increased almost perfectly in-line with seed oil consumption!

Thankfully medical interventions like stents have flattened the death rates of CVD slightly in recent years, but not the incidents of heart disease.

So, just to re-cap.

Vegetable/seed oils were not part of the diet before 1910 and heart disease didn't really exist (at least not noticeably) in Western civilisation until 1910-ish, deaths from heart disease and consumption of vegetable oil show almost perfect correlation in development for a century since then.

Now let's be clear.

This shows correlation, not causation.

What I mean by this is that, the correlation shows a matching trend, but it doesn't provide absolute, cast-iron proof that vegetable oil is single-handedly responsible for all heart disease deaths.

But with our knowledge of the pro-inflammatory effects of vegetable oils that shows them as a leading cause of oxidation, and our understanding that inflammation and oxidation are the drivers of heart disease, there is significant evidence to implicate vegetable oil consumption as a key contributor to our increasingly poor heart health.

Unlike natural saturated fats, such as lard, butter, tallow & coconut, vegetable oils are terrible for cooking with as they degrade and oxidise, creating reactive oxygen species that wreak-havoc with our health.

Seed oils are referred to as "vegetable" oils (probably to make them sound healthy).

Vegetable oils mainly come from the seeds of plants, many of which don't form part of the human diet, such as sunflower, rape, safflower and even cotton.

When was the last time you considered cotton a food?

Vegetable oil consumption is one of the few diet and lifestyle trends that has increased consistently in line with increasing rates of chronic disease.

In data from the Sydney Diet Heart Study[32], it was concluded that *"Substituting dietary linoleic acid in place of saturated fats increased the rates of death from all causes, coronary heart disease, and cardiovascular disease."*

When comparing heart disease death rates from a variety of factors this 7-year study concluded that *smoking a pack of cigarettes per day increases risk of death by 80%, whereas increasing vegetable oil consumption (by just 12% of calories) increases risk of death by 62%!*

So every 5% increase in daily calories from vegetable oil is as dangerous as smoking 7 cigarettes per day.

Another way of looking at it; each additional teaspoon of vegetable oil you consume could increase your risk of death as much as smoking 2 cigarettes.

In the MARGARIN study, 282 participants were separated into different groups and told to eat different types of margarine, either margarine made with more fat from vegetable oil or margarine made with less fat from vegetable oil.

After two years, the number of strokes, heart attacks and cardiovascular deaths was *seven times higher* in the group eating the vegetable oil rich margarine than in the group eating the margarine made with less vegetable oil.

Vegetable oils degrade from a molecular standpoint once heated, making them extremely dangerous to our bodies when used to cook with, but this is one of the main uses for them.

So which fats should you cook with?

---

32   https://www.bmj.com/content/346/bmj.e8707

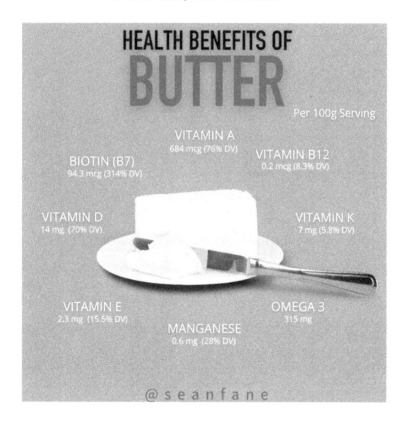

When cooking with a high heat, you should use oils that are stable and don't oxidise easily.

Nina Teicholz explains in *The Big Fat Surprise*;

"An oxidation product called 4-hydroxynonenal (HNE) was identified in the 1990s. This is an aldehyde. These are responsible for interfering with DNA and RNA and disturbing basic cell functioning. HNE's are produced by a number of vegetable oils at temperatures well below those regularly used for frying and below those at which the oils start to smoke or smell. HNE's are involved in atherosclerosis.

HNE's cause cholesterol to oxidise. HNE's reliably create oxidative stress in the body."

When oils undergo heat exposure they oxidise and form free-radicals and harmful compounds that you would do best to avoid.

All fats and oils are a combination of a variety of types of fatty acid, and the relative degree of saturation of fatty acids in an oil will determine its susceptibility to oxidation.

The more saturated the better, for reduced oxidation.

This is because saturated fats have single bonds but monounsaturated fats have one double bond and polyunsaturated fats have two or more double bonds, and it is these double bonds that are chemically reactive with heat, and break-down and become oxidised.

For these reasons saturated fats and monounsaturated fats are pretty resistant to oxidation from heating, but oils that are high in polyunsaturated fats should be avoided for cooking.

The best three fats for cooking then are:

Coconut Oil - Containing:

Saturated: 92%, Monounsaturated: 6%, Polyunsaturated: 1.6%

Butter - Containing:

Saturated: 68%, Monounsaturated: 28%, Polyunsaturated: 4%

Olive Oil - Containing:

Saturated: 14%, Monounsaturated: 75%, Polyunsaturated: 11%

Lard would have made it into the top 3, but the proportion of fatty acid varies a fair bit depending on the food the animal ate during its lifetime, so it is a variable that is tough to define specifically, but generally would be up alongside butter.

So you can see, that even the Mediterranean diet oil of choice, olive oil, is actually more prone to oxidation through heat than saturated fat, and isn't the heart-healthy choice. Maybe good to drizzle on a salad, but not the first choice to fry with.

What should you **NEVER** cook with?

Vegetable/seed oils such as; soybean oil, corn oil, cottonseed oil, canola oil, rapeseed oil, sunflower oil, sesame oil, grapeseed oil, safflower oil, rice bran oil.

The list seems endless these days.

If their standard make-up wasn't bad enough, seed oils have been shown to have up to 4% **trans fats** in their make-up [33]....the **Franken-Fat** of all terrible fats.

---

[33] https://onlinelibrary.wiley.com/doi/abs/10.1111/j.1745-4522.1994.tb00244.x

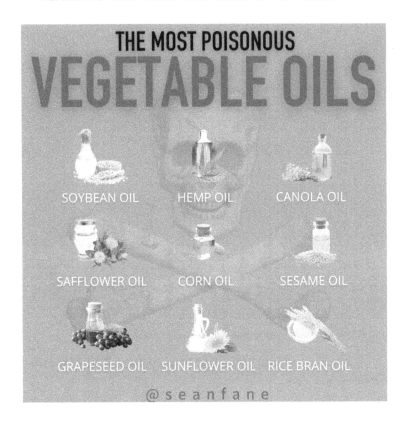

Seriously, if you have any of these oils in any cupboard anywhere, my advice would be to throw them away immediately.

You may wonder how industrial plants even get the oil out of some of these seeds…..which is actually a really good question!

Hexane is used in the oil extraction process.

Hexane is a chemical that is itself extracted from petroleum and crude oil. It is a colourless liquid that gives off a subtle, gasoline-like odour. Nice!

"Why use hexane to extract oil from seeds?" I hear you ask!

According to Pure Chemicals Group's website, hexane is preferred to pressing and other extraction methods because it provides:

- Maximum oil recovery

- Lesser working cost

- Cheaper price tags for end users

- Production meets demand

- The extracted oil is low in sedimentation

- Solvent loss is low

Doesn't sound like quality, safety or health are high on the list of reasons for choosing hexane as an extraction method does it?

Even short-term exposure to hexane [34] can cause damage to the human nervous system, unconsciousness, headaches and nausea.

In the MDS Online article **Understanding The Hazards of Hexane** they state;

"Because of its potential dangers, it is important to know how to handle and store this chemical properly and what to do in the unfortunate event of human exposure."

It is estimated that some hexane is still present in the final vegetable oil product that we pour out of our bottles.

In a 2017 study called **Evaluation of Hexane Content in Edible Vegetable Oils Consumed in Iran**, forty samples of different

---

[34] https://www.msdsonline.com/2014/11/19/understanding-the-hazards-of-hexane/

types of vegetable oil including frying, blended, sunflower, corn, and canola oils were investigated.

Hexane residue was detected in thirty-six out of forty examined samples.

Because of the way these oils are sneakily added to almost all processed foods our consumption of hidden vegetable oils is frighteningly high.

Some vegetable/seed oils are also bleached to make them look light and healthy, as they don't look quite so appealing otherwise.

So after heat and hexane and emulsification and bleach and sometimes synthetic colours, your cotton/sunflower/safflower seeds have now produced a lovely bottle of poison-containing, pro-inflammatory oil that will break-down under heat exposure when you cook with it, to make it even more toxic.

Hard to understand why this has replaced butter in baked goods and for cooking isn't it!

Other than the fact that there is a massive agricultural industry that operates by providing these cheap vegetable oils to industry, and has created the propaganda that they are "heart healthy".

Even more ironic that where America went, with regards to eating seed oil, the rest of the developed world duly followed, and the advice of the American Heart Association, and the USA government guidelines, stretched all the way from the United States to the rest of the Western world as a manifesto for good health.

Whilst these same countries all struggled with an explosion of modern chronic disease, an enormous industry for the huge amount of crops grown in the United States developed.

These oils were heavily promoted as "heart healthy" from the early 1970's. Look at the advert below.

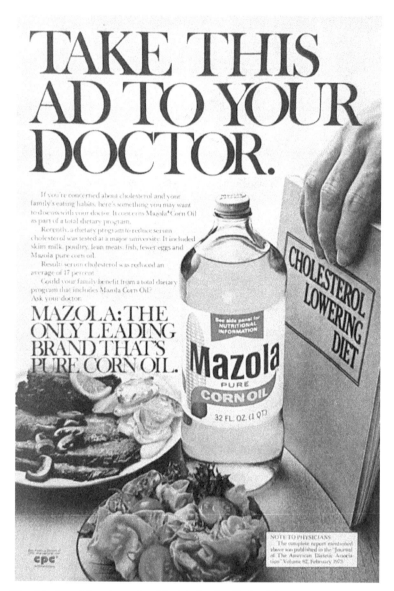

The National Institute for Health in the United States even spent hundreds of millions of dollars in the 1960's and 1970's trying to prove that vegetable oils were healthy, in order to solidify their position as our primary choice for consumption, and had enlisted the support of experts Ancel Keys and Jerry Stamler.

These were the very people that had already demonised saturated fat, so they could be relied upon to promote the alternative choice of vegetable oil consumption.

As Nina Teicholz describes in her book *The Big Fat Surprise* one such trial designed to prove the health benefits of vegetable oils was called MR FIT (Multiple Risk Factor Intervention Trial) and ran from 1973 to 1982, and as she puts it *"Was one of the biggest and most demanding medical experiments ever performed on a group of human beings, involving 28 medical centres nationwide at a cost of $115 million."*

The study measured 361,000 middle aged men and found 12,000 whose cholesterol was 290 mg/dL…what they considered *"so high that they were at imminent risk of a heart attack."*

Most of these were obese, smokers, with high blood-pressure and plenty of other risk-factors.

The aim of the study was to promote vegetable oils as an alternative to saturated fat. *NB (The aim of any study is supposed to be to understand the evidence, not for it to prove an existing view that helps the business interests of the funders.....but never mind).*

Half of this sub-group was given every intervention known at the time to improve heart health from counselling for stress, to blood-pressure lowering medication, exercise plans and a diet of skimmed milk, *margarine*, limited eggs to two per week or less, no butter, no meat, *less than 8% of their diet to come from saturated fat.* (it was replaced with fats from vegetable oils).

The other half of the sub-group was told to do whatever they liked, so they carried on with the lifestyles that had created their very poor heart health in the first place, and were left to fend for themselves.

7 years later the results were in.

Unfortunately for the study organisers, desperate to show that saturated fat was bad for health and vegetable oils were not (which was the whole basis for the experiment in the first place) *the men in the intervention group died at higher rates than the group of men that didn't change their diet and lifestyles at all.*

Even worse, the 16 year follow-up of the study confirmed a higher degree of lung cancer in the intervention group, even though 21% of them had quit smoking compared to the 6% that had in the control group.

Oops!

There seemed to be a bit of a problem here then.

I think we can agree that the counselling, reduced smoking, increased exercise and lowered blood pressure from medications are unlikely to have been the things that contributed to a higher death rate in the intervention group….so what does that leave us with?

It leaves the swap of saturated fat to vegetable oil.

Not only were deaths increased but so were incidences of cancer, from the group that swapped saturated fat for vegetable oils…..despite all of the other positive lifestyle adaptations that this group were given!

Pretty damning results for vegetable oils, I am sure you will agree.

Astonishingly, as Teicholz explains in her book, despite the terrible results, the trial organisers continued to ignore the *elephant in the room* and instead, they promoted *cherry-picked* elements of the data in order to try to reinforce their pre-trial, biased view that saturated fat was bad and that vegetable oils were not.

This kind of biased research and cherry-picked data, based on vested interests funding research still continues in some trials today.

In fact most of the demonisation of saturated fat and promotion of vegetable oils is based on manipulated data from corporate vested interests, that fund much of the research.

In his book ***Doctoring Data*** Dr Malcolm Kendrick explains the many ways in which this kind of medical "hood-winking" has become so prevalent in the defence of biased views related to health policy over the years.

So, now that I have made my case against them, what afflictions will befall you from consuming seed oils?

Well, pretty much every chronic inflammatory condition is caused, or exacerbated, by this kind of toxic substance, including heart disease, insulin resistance and even dementia.

Canola oil is a great example of an oil described as healthy, and looking at its Omega 3 to Omega 6 ratios you could be forgiven for thinking it may be a good choice (even if you ignore all the processing issues). But it isn't.

According to BulletProof.com:

Canola oil looks like an optimal vegetable-based oil, with a healthy 2:1 ratio of omega-6 to omega-3 fatty acids, and ideally, you want all of the foods you consume to have an omega-6 to omega-3 ratio in the neighbourhood of 4:1 or less.

However, the omega-6 to omega-3 fatty acid ratio of 2:1 comes in the form of short-chain alpha linoleic acid (ALA). To use short-chain ALA fatty acids, the human body must first convert ALA to the long-chain fatty acids (EPA) and (DHA) before it can be used.

Unfortunately, ALA converts to EPA at a rate of about 5%, and converts to DHA at a rate of less than 1%. What this means is that the 2:1 ratio isn't accurate. Less than 6% of the omega-3s can be used by the body, making the ratio closer to 8:1 which is not good!

To re-cap then, the oils www.bulletproof.com recommend for cooking and eating for optimum health are shown in the picture below:

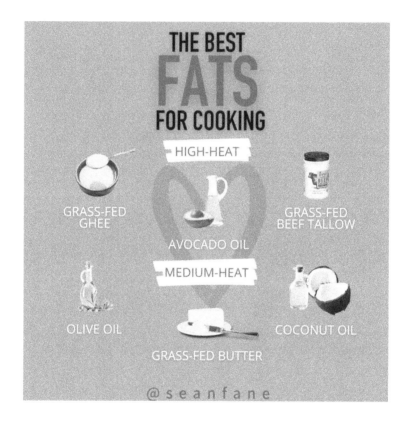

When you aren't cooking, use extra virgin olive oil and walnut oil for salad dressings.

LIFESTYLE

Nan's Chapter Summary: Your lifestyle choices can dramatically affect your heart-health.

Smoking is one of the biggest risk factors in ones lifestyle for heart disease.

There aren't many things you can do worse than smoking to directly introduce harmful chemicals into your body, to create the inflammation that leads to CVD.

Being generally active can be under-rated, and is a significant aspect of good health.

Whilst it doesn't really feel like exercise, being on your feet and engaged in movement is extremely important to keep your muscles and bones strong, and also to improve your hormone balance.

Don't sit for too long before getting-up and enjoying some movement.

Loneliness and isolation increase stress, and these can lead to hormone imbalances that damage your heart health.

It is important to stay connected to your friends and family.

Good sleep is very important for hormone balance, and to help you manage your blood sugar levels.

Try to go to bed and wake-up at a regular time to ensure that you get a good night's sleep.

After food, the aspect of your health where you can exert the most control is your lifestyle.

We all get into habits over the years that cumulatively create either positive impacts or negative impacts on our health, relationships and life.

These habits can also, over time, accelerate and promote chronic disease, or decelerate and prevent chronic disease.

Smoking

This is a biggie!

Smoking is pretty much the mother of all inflammatory evils.

Smoking is essentially the act of taking harmful toxic compounds directly into your bloodstream via your lungs.

Cigarettes, cigars, and pipe tobacco are made from dried tobacco leaves, but other substances are added for flavour and to make smoking more pleasant (like sugar for example, which has been added to tobacco leaves for over a century to facilitate the ability to inhale more smoke).

The smoke inhaled is a damaging mixture of chemicals from burning the tobacco and the additives from the manufacturing process.

Tobacco smoke is made up of thousands of chemicals, with at least 70 known to be carcinogenic.

Some of the chemicals found in tobacco smoke include:

- Hydrogen cyanide

- Formaldehyde

- Lead

- Arsenic

- Ammonia

- Radioactive elements, such as polonium-210

- Benzene

- Carbon Monoxide

- Tobacco-Specific Nitrosamines (TSNAs)

- Polycyclic Aromatic Hydrocarbons (PAHs)

Many of these substances heavily contribute to heart disease, lung disease, or other serious health problems.

"Cigarette smoke causes considerable morbidity and mortality by inducing cancer, chronic lung and vascular diseases, and oral disease. Despite the well-recognized risks associated with smoking, the habit remains unacceptably prevalent. " was the conclusion of the scholarly article titled *Cigarette Smoking & Inflammation* [35] published in 2011 by J Lee et al. which described the mechanisms for inflammation derived from cigarette smoke.

Even passive smoking, the act of breathing the exhaled residue from the air surrounding a smoker is a big issue.

A serum cotinine test is usually the most reliable way to evaluate tobacco use, or exposure to tobacco smoke, because it is a substance that is only produced when nicotine is metabolised.

In a US health and nutritional examination survey [36] conducted between 1998 and 1991 it was discovered that in non-tobacco users (non-smokers) *"87.9% had detectable levels of serum cotinine, which indicated that these groups had higher exposure to environmental tobacco smoke".*

So nearly 90% of non-smokers have the evidence of inhaled toxins from cigarette smoke.

Does this mean passive smoking is also a heart health risk?

---

[35] https://www.ncbi.nlm.nih.gov/pmc/articles/PMC3261116/

[36] https://pubmed.ncbi.nlm.nih.gov/8601954/

In *Passive Smoking and the Risk of Coronary Heart Disease* [37] Jiang He, M.D et al. performed a meta-analysis of epidemiological studies by examining the Medline database (from January 1966 through June 1998) for literature with the medical subject headings "tobacco smoke pollution," "coronary disease," and "myocardial infarction" and the key words "passive smoking" and "environmental tobacco smoke."

They also conducted a search of abstracts listed in *Dissertation Abstracts Online* using the key word "passive smoking," and performed a manual search of references cited in published original and review articles.

They stated

"Active cigarette smoking is one of the most important modifiable risk factors for coronary heart disease". And also concluded that *"Passive smoking is associated with a small increase in the risk of coronary heart disease."*

"Because of the high prevalence of passive cigarette smoking at home and in the workplace, a substantial number of coronary events occur, with implications for public health."

So yes, even passive smoking increases our risk for heart disease.

Smoking also accelerates insulin resistance, the foundation of all metabolic health issues.

As Ben Bikman writes in Why We Get Sick;

---

[37]   https://www.nejm.org/doi/full/10.1056/nejm199903253401204

"Work from my laboratory has identified that even secondhand smoke is enough to produce ceramides, the main drivers of smoke-induced insulin resistance."

Interestingly, studies have shown that smoking has a greater negative impact on women than men.

Although women and men share most classic risk factors, the significance and the relative weighting of these factors are different. At younger ages (less than 50 years old) smoking is more deleterious to women than men, with a larger negative impact of the total number of cigarettes smoked per day.

In young pre-menopausal women, smoking causes a reduction in the protective effect of oestrogen (which can help expansion of artery walls).

If you smoke you increase your risk of heart disease regardless of whichever other risk factors are present or absent.

If preventing inflammation is a goal, then smoking cigarettes is the epitome of poor practice.

Sitting

I remember receiving a jibe from an Australian spectator during the coverage of a recent Olympic Games.

After cheering home a win for Ben Ainslie in the sailing event, the chap, obviously annoyed that I was so pleased suggested that the British were lazy as a nation.

When asked what he meant by that he replied that "Even at the Olympics, you only get medals for sports where you're sitting down!"

I checked the medals table for Great Britain, and annoyingly he had a point, which did make me laugh a bit.

The GB team had medals for sailing, rowing, cycling and show-jumping at the time.

Joking aside though we all spend too much of our time sitting down.

Being sedentary is not really the act of *doing something* to create heart disease risk.

It is the act of doing *nothing*.....to create heart disease risk.

Our heart is a muscle, designed to work 24 hours a day, 365 days a year until we die, but like a car that is designed to be driven, it doesn't like being left idle for long periods of time.

Atrophy, where muscles decrease in size and strength through lack of use, is a significant enemy of good health. Our heart is a muscle, and it will atrophy to a point from lack of use, along with our other muscles.

Hypertrophy is the opposite, where muscles grow stronger through exercise and recovery.

Whether we want to build big 'guns', or have 'washboard'-abs, or just have better strength for our daily lives, we can exercise our muscles in order that they can perform well and stay strong.

Our heart receives exercise from everything that we do that encourages movement throughout the other muscles in our body, as the muscles we use need energy and oxygen delivered to them to keep them contracting, so our heart beats faster to pump more blood into them.

The less muscles we engage, and the lower the intensity level of contraction, the less our heart works to feed them and provide energy.

The more muscles we engage, and the greater the intensity level of contraction, the more our heart works to feed them and provide energy.

Whilst doing too much exercise, too intensely, with a heart condition should be taken under advice, walking is a great activity that strengthens the heart but isn't too strenuous for most people to do.

If we have the ability to track our activity through a step-counter, mobile phone or watch (after a heart attack in the UK you will be given one for this purpose anyway) and if we don't already engage in at least 10,000 steps a day and keep active, we should. It keeps our hearts healthy and strong. This equates to about an hour and a half of brisk walking per day.

A strong heart may still suffer from a heart attack, but it is far more likely to escape unscathed from a minor event, or recover more quickly afterwards from something more serious.

Sitting really does switch all muscular activity off, and we sit for most of our waking day, whether in the car, at a table to eat, in the office or resting at home.

I like to create little life-hacks to break this cycle of inactivity.

Every 15 minutes that I sit at my desk I get up and walk around the house, or make a cup of tea, or just do some standing squats in my office.

If I receive or make a mobile phone call I do it whilst standing and walking....it is a *mobile* phone after all.

I have placed a pair of dumbbells at the door of my utility room, and a yoga mat in the shower room.

Each time I go to take a shower or let the dogs out, I am reminded to do a few sit-ups or dumbbell exercises.

It doesn't need to be much and I don't need a gym membership, or to get hot and sweaty, but these are tiny little reminders for me to keep moving and active, and they help to wake my heart-up from its inactivity.

All of these things help to counter-act the negative consequences of sitting down.

If you feel that you have a lifestyle where you spend a lot of time sitting it may be worth thinking about little things that you can do to break this up and create small moments of activity throughout your day.

Lack Of Connection

Loneliness is the new smoking!

Everything from anxiety, depression, anger, fear and heartbreak can trigger the stress hormones that will negatively impact your wellbeing and your heart health.

Being lonely is damaging, yet I get the feeling that it is not considered quite as serious by the general public as something that expresses itself more physically.

In the study *Women, Loneliness, and Incident Coronary Heart Disease*[38] from 2009, it was shown that loneliness was associated with increased risk of incident coronary heart disease amongst women.

The authors concluded;

"Loneliness was prospectively associated with increased risk of incident CHD, controlling for multiple confounding factors. Loneliness among women may merit clinical attention, not only due to its impact on quality of life but also its potential implications for cardiovascular health."

In a 2016 meta-analysis entitled *Loneliness and social isolation as risk factors for coronary heart disease and stroke*[39] the authors concluded;

"Our findings suggest that deficiencies in social relationships are associated with an increased risk of developing CHD and stroke. Future studies are needed to investigate

---

[38]   https://www.ncbi.nlm.nih.gov/pmc/articles/PMC2851545/

[39]   https://heart.bmj.com/content/102/13/1009.short

whether interventions targeting loneliness and social isola-tion can help to prevent two of the leading causes of death and disability in high-income countries. "

Throughout this book the impact of mental health on our physical health will be examined, and some strategies for improving mental health will be explored, but social connection is a fundamental element of great mental health, and it is something we should all prioritise. Not just because it is great to see and speak with our family and friends, but because it is good for us too.

When I was a volunteer for The Samaritans, I would receive calls from people that were desperate and suicidal, and many with mental health issues, but the majority of the calls were from people that were very lonely and didn't have anybody to talk to.

Loneliness is a common feature of our modern lives, and we should work pro-actively to reduce its health impacts on ourselves and our loved-ones by increasing our connection wherever we can.

Everybody should do what they can to prioritise social interaction for good health. Not doing so can increase the risk of heart disease.

Sleeplessness

It has been shown in a number of studies, that sleeplessness is casu-ally associated with heart disease.

It has been known for a long time that cortisol is elevated when sleep is disrupted, and when sleep is deprived. This may be one factor at play.

Additionally, poor sleep and elevated cortisol can have the terrible knock-on consequence of elevating blood glucose, which in turn creates a need for insulin, which sets one up for a terrible cascade of hormonal turmoil.

In ***Causal Assessment Of Sleep On Coronary Heart Disease*** [40], researchers modelled data from a number of studies and concluded;

> *"Our analysis provided evidence supporting a causal relationship between sleeplessness and CHD."*

It is highly recommended that sleep becomes a key lifestyle priority, and that we form regular end-of-the-day habits to promote good sleep, in the same way that we have regular start-of-the-day habits like cleaning our teeth and having a shower.

---

[40]

https://www.sciencedirect.com/science/article/abs/pii/S13899457 19302953

WHY DO WE BELIEVE WHAT WE DO?

Nan's Chapter Summary: *In the 1950's a very ambitious man thought he had discovered a link between cholesterol and heart disease. He also pointed-out that saturated fat can raise cholesterol. When he published his discovery he received acclaim, and positions of power in the medical community and within the United States government, where he advised on public health guidelines.*

When other scientists and medical researchers highlighted that his theory about cholesterol was incorrect, he used his power and influence to discredit them, and to continue to assert that he was right. He didn't ever manage to create a trial to prove his theory, even though he spent the rest of his life trying to do so.

Despite this, the United States government, and the other large American companies that benefited from the replacement of fats and meat with grains and carbohydrates grown in America, continued to advise against saturated fats.

Over the remaining years, other large organisations, like the pharmaceutical companies that make cholesterol lowering drugs, have spent hundreds of millions of dollars on advertising, lobbying and studies trying to maintain the belief that cholesterol is bad, because they make a lot of money selling drugs to lower cholesterol

So if cholesterol is essential for life, and all cholesterol is so good for us....why the hell has it generated such a bad reputation over the years?

Good question!

I won't go into too much detail here because it is a very long and detailed story, best told by authors like Nina Teicholz in her amazing book ***The Big Fat Surprise***.

To cut a long story short, in the 1950's a very influential and ambitious physiologist called Ancel Keys created a hypothesis that saturated fat was responsible for heart disease, because it raises cholesterol.

He provided a plausible explanation of associations, for an expectant public, not long after the US President had suffered a heart-attack.

He took some weak data that showed some correlation (not the same as showing cause) and extrapolated this into a theory that saturated fat caused heart disease.

Ironically, his work was funded by many different lobby groups that supported the sugar industries and agriculture in the US, so any similar correlations (which were proven to be more likely) between sugar or carbohydrates and heart disease were ignored, in fact even buried.

His hypothesis seemed reasonable to many in the medical community in the United States at the time, and soon the agricultural industry & commercial sugar associations threw their considerable political and financial weight behind his ideas.

Of course if fat and meat were bad for heart health, then people would switch to eating more cereals, grains and products containing sugar, which was good for their businesses.

Keys and his advocates went on to advise and head-up some of the formal associations that created law and health guidelines in America over the years.

Soon the pharmaceutical industry, becoming more powerful through treating heart disease and lowering cholesterol, became involved in funding research to support this concept of heart disease which became known as the ***cholesterol hypothesis***, or the ***diet heart hypothesis***.

These organisations profit from sugar, crops, drugs and medical supplies.

Their financial interests are aligned, and are best served selling the foods that create bad health and then selling the drugs to treat the resulting medical conditions.

Everybody profits!

It sounds like some terrible Machiavellian plot, but in reality it was just a bad idea that some financial institutions took advantage of, and have done for many years since.

Back to Ancel Keys and his diet heart hypothesis…..

Keys "doubled-down" on this position regarding saturated fat over the years, despite evidence demonstrating his logic and science was flawed.

Growing numbers in the medical and research communities understood he was wrong, but eventually the ***Seven Countries Study (A Keys study)*** was held-up as the final justification for Key's hypothesis to become governmental health policy in the USA.

The rest of the Western world has followed suit and adopted the US recommendations for heart-health advice ever since.

The Seven Countries Study was Keys' "cherry-picked" data, supporting his hypothesis, and the evidence did not support its conclusions, however we spent the next half a century in the misguided belief that saturated fat causes heart disease.

Nina Teicholz points out some of the bias and data omissions relating to the Seven Countries Study in her book;

*"**There were some vexing problems with data points that failed to support his hypothesis. Eastern Finns died of heart disease at rates three times that of western Finns, yet their lifestyles and diets, according to Keys' data, were virtually identical. The islanders of Corfu ate even less saturated fat than did their countrymen on Crete, yet on Corfu rates of heart disease were far higher. Thus, within countries, the***

correlation between saturated fat and heart disease didn't hold-up."

"In the study the people that lived the longest overall lived in Greece and the United States, and their longevity showed no relationship to the amount of fat or saturated fat they ate, nor the cholesterol levels in their blood."

And of one particular part of the study Teicholz noted;

"Of the 12,770 participants, the food they ate was only evaluated for 499 of them (3.9%)."

Keys actually studied 21 countries, and had selected the 7 countries that were most likely to support his hypothesis.

Subsequent research of the data from all 21 countries from his research shows **no correlation between saturated fat and heart disease**, and yet Keys managed to assert the opposite, and garner the fierce support of the large American institutions that benefited from the outcomes.

Even to this day, despite the western world continuing to follow the guidelines created from this massive deception, this belief is still known as the "diet heart **hypothesis**" because despite hundreds of millions of pounds being poured into research to **try** to prove a link between saturated fat and heart disease, none has ever been demonstrated.

In his 2016 book **The Case Against Sugar**, Gary Taubes noted about the Seven Countries Study that;

"Of all the factors measured in these populations, the two that tracked best with heart disease were sugar and saturated fat and because populations in the study that ate a lot of one tended also to eat a lot of the other, Keys suggested that this was adequate to explain the observed relationship between saturated fat and heart disease without recourse to the idea that sucrose caused it."

The *French Paradox* was often brought up when scientists debated the role of saturated fat in heart disease.

For many years it has been noted that when charts of the highest saturated fat consumption in Europe are compiled, the French and the Swiss invariably feature at the top of the charts. You probably could have guessed that, with all the butter and cream and meat that goes into traditional French cuisine.

So I guess they must be falling-down in the streets of Paris riddled with chronic heart-disease right?

When the analysis of heart attack deaths for Europe were examined for the same periods as the saturated fat consumption, paradoxically, the French and the Swiss are at the bottom.

They have the highest saturated fat consumption, but the lowest heart-disease!

Clearly, if one is to believe that saturated fats are the cause of heart disease, one must first disregard all of the data and evidence ever collected on the subject, which entirely disproves this false belief.

The WHO MONICA project[41] is a programme that focuses on trends in event rates for validated fatal and non-fatal coronary heart attacks and strokes.

In 2009 they noted:

Average cholesterol in men in Russia was 5.1 mol/l. CHD deaths per 100,000 in Russia were 267 per 100,000.

---

[41]   https://pubmed.ncbi.nlm.nih.gov/3335877/

Average cholesterol in men in Switzerland it was 6.4 mmol/l. CHD deaths per 100,000 in Switzerland were 32 per 100,000.

Patty Siri-Tarino PhD, Ronald Krauss MD of the Children's Hospital Oakland Research Institute & Frank B Hu of Harvard performed a meta-analysis[42] of the effect of saturated fat on heart disease.

21 studies qualified for inclusion. 347,747 subjects had been followed and their diets analysed for between 5 and 23 years. 11,006 of these developed Coronary Heart Disease or strokes.

The meta-analysis concluded:

"Intake of saturated fat was not associated with an increased risk of Coronary Heart Disease or stroke, nor was it associated with an increased risk of Cardio Vascular Disease."

So I hope you now understand what categorically doesn't cause heart disease.

As Nina Teicholz writes;

"After the diet-heart hypothesis became adopted by the AHA and the NIH, Key's bias was institutionalised!"

In fact the bias got nailed into a financial gravy-train that hasn't stopped accelerating since.

Teicholz continues;

"The American Heart Association, in the 1960s, decided that heart disease is caused by saturated fat in the diet and the men at high risk of heart disease should eat little of it."

---

[42] https://pubmed.ncbi.nlm.nih.gov/20071648/

"This flawed and misleading health advice continued despite the persistent failure of any clinical trials to actually confirm this hypothesis".

Even the American Heart Association, one of the organisations most to blame for perpetuating the myth that saturated fat causes heart disease, is quietly changing its message now though.

They have recently conceded, after 50 years of saying the opposite:

"In the Women's Health Initiative randomised clinical trial, a reduction of total fat consumption from 37.8% of energy to 24.3% of energy had no effect on Coronary Heart Disease, Stroke or total CVD."

They have also confirmed (after pooled analysis from 11 cohort studies covering 344,696 participants) that;

"Each 5% higher energy consumption of carbohydrates in place of saturated fat was associated with a 7% higher risk of cardiovascular disease".

Further to an act passed in 1992, The FDA (Food & Drug Administration) in America gets paid a fee on all pharmaceutical drugs sold.

The FDA describes themselves as;

"Responsible for protecting the public health by ensuring the safety, efficacy, and security of human and veterinary drugs, biological products, and medical devices; and by ensuring the safety of our nation's food supply, cosmetics, and products that emit radiation."

So, in essence, the regulatory body for drug acceptance gets paid a percentage of drug sales....it in fact receives more than $300m a year.

So not much incentive to reduce drug use there then!!

In fact, the more drugs sold to deal with the issues created through bad food choices, the more money the FDA generates for itself.

Genius!

If ever there was a more blatant example from a public health perspective, of a fox guarding the hen-house, I can't think of one.

What even *is* high cholesterol?

Above 5 mmol/l in the UK...above 5.2 mmol/l in the US (200mg/dl) and above 4 mmol/l in anyone who has suffered heart attack or stroke is considered high cholesterol.

This was decreed at the US National Cholesterol Consensus Conference in 1984....with no evidence to support the levels ...chosen....just numbers plucked arbitrarily, seemingly from thin-air.

Malcolm Kendrick - A Statin Nation explains;

"70% of the western world is above this "normal" threshold....and as our average cholesterol decreases with statin use...and heart disease increases rapidly alongside it...the target numbers are pushed lower and lower....until I guess they are zero."

"Then I guess we will have epidemic levels of CVD, no cholesterol at all, and a completely sick society".

"At this point I guess the penny will drop with the medical community that they were the judge that convicted the innocent man!"

One last word on cholesterol, as you may read articles from well-meaning, but mis-informed people, claiming that eating more plant-based products will lower your cholesterol.

This, as I have mentioned is not a good thing.

A quote from the Journal of Biological Sciences:

"It is widely accepted that cholesterol lowering is helpful per se. We challenge this view, with particular reference to plant sterols. Cholesterol lowering should not be an end

148

in itself. The objective must be to reduce outcomes, such as incidence of coronary heart disease. We hypothesised that plant sterols may lower cholesterol, but not coronary heart disease. We found the outcome on coronary heart disease in fact to be detrimental."

WHY DOESN'T MY DOCTOR KNOW THIS?

Nan's Chapter Summary: *Statins are medication given to us to lower cholesterol.*

I hope you understand what a bad idea that is by this stage of the book!

Statins have been proven to cause many dangerous side effects including increasing diabetes and accelerating dementia and even causing heart attacks, but they have not been proven to save lives or improve CVD outcomes".

If you decide to take statins, you should be fully aware of the risks, which include potential memory loss, muscle weakness, impotence and kidney problems.

Speak with your doctor, if you are prescribed statins, and make sure you ask him to explain all the potential issues, and always make him aware if you experience any side effects.

In *Statins Should Not Be Given To Patients With Heart Failure!* [43] the effect of Rosuvastatin was measured in patients with chronic heart failure.

The results are outlined in the pictorial below.

---

[43]   https://pubmed.ncbi.nlm.nih.gov/18757089/

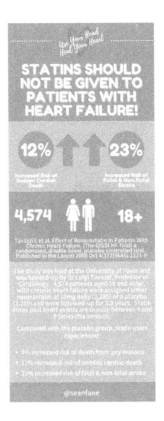

Those taking the statin has a slightly higher death-rate overall, 12% increased risk of sudden cardiac death and a 23% increased risk of stroke, even though the doses of statin used were much lower than are normally prescribed for most patients.

When I had started to understand the scientific data relating to statins, I really had to wrestle with my conflicting feelings on what to do for myself, because the scientific evidence goes entirely against the mainstream advice from medical professionals.

I had been prescribed the highest dose of Atorvastatin straight from hospital, after my PCI was performed and the stent was fitted, no explanation, no discussion, just a prescription handed to me as I left the ward.

Some time during the first year of post heart-attack recovery I had read enough to convince me that I should stop taking statins, and I had told my doctor that I had done so when I next saw them.

Soon after I had been asked to come and see my GP, as I had explained to them the last time I was in for a check-up that I wasn't taking my statins, and they were not happy.

At the time, I didn't realise that GP's were financially incentivised to ensure adherence to taking certain drugs in the UK, so I thought their insistence on seeing me again to convince me to start taking them was just a mis-placed concern for my health. Maybe it was.

When I eventually visited my doctor, ready for the "telling-off" I was about to receive for refusing to take my statins, I had 4 questions prepared for him, and I decided that if he answered them all to my satisfaction, and had some compelling data to change my mind, that I might re-consider the statins.

The questions were:

1. Do you know what the mevalonate pathway[44] is and what it does?

2. If cholesterol is so bad for our health, why is it prioritised by the liver for production?

3. Do you know of any clinical trials that have shown that saturated fat and cholesterol cause heart disease?

4. What is the efficacy, and what are the potential side effects of statins?

---

44   https://en.wikipedia.org/wiki/Mevalonate_pathway

When I arrived, I was told my GP was away and had been replaced by another at the practice, and she started off by asking me to sit, before checking her notes and diving straight in. (The following is para-phrased as I did not record the exact words used in the conversation);

"Why aren't you taking your statins? It is vitally important that we lower your cholesterol because it is too high!"

My LDL had increased slightly since I had changed my diet to eat more saturated fat, and was now at the upper end of "normal".

I went straight-in too!

"Thanks for inviting me in. I have been doing a lot of reading on statins and cholesterol and I wanted to ask you a few questions because the information I have read seems a little confusing." I started.

First question….

"Do you know what the mevalonate pathway is and what it does?"

Answer: "No!"

My response: "Oh. OK. It is the 37-step process that our bodies undertake to create cholesterol along with many other substances important to life. Statins interrupt this pathway so early in the process that they inhibit the production of Co-Enzyme Q10, which is important for muscle function, including the function of the heart muscle. This, statin-interrupted, pathway is the cornerstone of the production of sex hormones, anabolic hormones, bile and vitamin D."

She looked a little dumbstruck!

"Oh. Well all I can say is that we have brought you in here to take statins because you are at high-risk and we need to reduce your cholesterol to reduce your risk of another heart attack!"

In I went with question 2.

"Ah, OK. If cholesterol is so bad for our health, why is it prioritised by the liver for production?"

"Look, you have clearly done some research, but we have protocols to follow and one of them is to protect patients from heart disease by encouraging them to take statins, so that's all I am trying to do."

Question 3 didn't get answered either.

"Do you know of any clinical trials that have shown that saturated fat and cholesterol cause heart disease?"

At this point the barrier of doctor and patient came down, and we started to chat person to person.

She explained that GP's don't have time to keep-up with medical data and research.

She told me that I probably knew more about heart disease than 95% of GP's (and remember I had only asked her 3 questions and only responded to one at this stage) which is worrying.

She then proceeded to tell me a story about her brother-in-law, who was a super-fit ultra-marathon runner with no body-fat, great cholesterol readings (that meant low to her...although you and I now know that low is bad), never smoked and in his early 40's and had the year before suffered an unexpected heart attack.

Apparently he, like me, had also refused to take statins, had done some research and was eating a ketogenic diet and taking a few supplements, whilst searching for genetic issues and the underlying cause.

Hallelujah!

She even gave me his number and told me to get in-touch, she thought we might "collaborate on a book or something".

Her parting comments, as I left the practice, were that so many of the beliefs pertaining to heart health have changed, and that the medical community is generally very slow to adapt to these changes because they are driven by the protocols that they are taught, and paid, to administer.

Now I tell you this anecdote, for no other reason than to show, that with very little interrogation, and a small amount of information at your fingertips, your GP may well perform a complete U-turn from insisting that you take statins to accepting that you won't.

How can it be so easy to destroy the framework of medical advice for a fatal condition?

I want my doctor to either, know definitively what is best for me, or refer me to a specialist that does.

I don't want them to insist on medicating me with something that might damage my health and accelerate a terminal condition, when they don't understand my underlying condition or the effects of what they are prescribing.

To prescribe a statin, which not only *doesn't* prevent heart disease, but makes it worse, is totally unconscionable in my view.

It is unfathomable to me how this is allowed to continue.

There is barely a doctor in the world that hasn't been trained to administer statins after every heart attack, stroke or diagnosis of type 2 diabetes.

Doctors are prescribing statins as a matter of course in some cases just as a precaution and with no symptoms of any of the above conditions when men reach 60.

There has been much debate about the prescription of statins for many years, but evaluation of the independent clinical trials and studies highlight a few facts worth knowing.

- There is **NO** general reduction in mortality rates for heart disease in those taking statins

- There is **INCREASED MORTALITY** from "all causes" in those taking statins (that means higher death rates)

- There are many side effects from taking statins, some of which are mild, some of which are life-destroying and others still which are terminal

- The only group of people that has been shown to derive any benefit from taking statins (and the benefit is eye-wateringly small) is specifically middle-aged men that have already had at least one heart attack. This group has shown a tiny improvement in incidences of a recurrent event, in one particular trial, which is believed to be from some of the anti-inflammatory effect that statins have.

- The small benefit derived from the sub-group above equates to circa 4.1 days of additional life extension from a heart attack after 5 continuous years of statin use (and that may require you living with some serious side effects for those 5 years and beyond).

To quote Dr Malcolm Kendrick in A Statin Nation;

"The Cochrane Collaboration, one of the only unbiased groups of researchers in the world, looked at SAE's (serious adverse events...like deaths from CHD and all other causes) from statin trials and found that total SAE's were unchanged by statins. To put it another way statins caused as many serious adverse events as they prevented (delayed). Or, to put it another way, they didn't do any bloody good!"

Once you are considered at high-risk for a heart attack by your doctor, you will be prescribed statins as a matter of course.

What your doctor considers high-risk, is a bar that is becoming lower and lower, year after year.

It includes some things that do increase your risk, such as men over 40 that are overweight, smoke or have diabetes.

It also, however, includes things like cholesterol levels, which don't increase your risk.

However, in either case, what the evidence shows is that statins do nothing to reduce death from cardiovascular disease or coronary heart disease, and this seems to have passed the medical community by.

The side effects are also generally washed under the carpet as insignificant by doctors.

I was advised by 4 doctors (that I subsequently asked the same questions as I asked my GP on the visit mentioned above) that they didn't know of any side effects of taking statins.

Given the research, and the number of community groups that discuss the life-altering impact of the side effects they have had, this is nothing short of mind-boggling!

For a little walk through some of the experiences of people who have had their lives wrecked by Statins, maybe head over to the Facebook Group called *Statins - The Silent Killer*[45] where currently over 5,000 members discuss the myriad of issues they have had with statin use (or any number of other forums which discuss the issues with statins).

Dr Kendrick explains again in A Statin Nation, how in recent history the medical community, and biased statin-funded research has falsified the details around the harmful effects of statins;

"Lets look at Cerivastatin. In 1997 this was one of the last of the statins to be unleashed on the public. It was, I think, the most potent at reducing LDL levels. This is what was written about it in a 1998 report called 'Cerivastatin in primary hyperlipidemia - a multicenter analysis of efficacy and safety':

---

45   https://www.facebook.com/groups/587055831344762/?ref=share

Cerivastatin is generally well tolerated and adverse effects have been mild and transient'. In 1998 the following was written about it: "The good tolerability made Cerivastatin a safe, well-tolerated and highly effective HMG-CoA reductase inhibitor'."

BUT......In 2001 it should be noted, just 3 years later, the following admission was announced "Cerivastatin was withdrawn from the market after 52 deaths attributed to drug-related rhabdomyolysis that lead to kidney failure!"

Not only is this all pretty damning for statins, more research has actually demonstrated that statins can **cause** and **exacerbate** heart disease.

In the study ***Statins Stimulate Atherosclerosis And Heart Failure!***[46] (catchy title) published in 2015, the authors concluded...

"In contrast to the current belief that cholesterol reduction with statins decreases atherosclerosis, we present a perspective that statins may be causative in coronary artery calcification through the depletion of coenzyme Q10 and 'heme A', and thereby ATP generation. Statins inhibit the synthesis of vitamin K2, which in turn protects arteries from calcification."

"The epidemic of heart failure and atherosclerosis that plagues the modern world may paradoxically be aggravated by the pervasive use of statin drugs. We propose that current statin treatment guidelines be critically re-evaluated."

---

[46]   https://pubmed.ncbi.nlm.nih.gov/25655639/

When you understand some of the sordid history of statins, their ubiquitous administration by doctors becomes even more shocking.

After 2005, when the EU adopted new regulations on reporting for clinical trials (to combat the "cherry-picking" of information that was crating very misleading conclusions from the research), statin trials have consistently failed to demonstrate any consistent mortality benefit, whereas before 2005, trials had espoused positive effects from statin treatment.

Very suspicious!

The number of individuals, in positions of power, that influenced the adoption and acceptance of these drugs *knowing* they were dangerous and -knowing *they aren't effective is staggering.*

A case in point.

Daniel Steinberg. If you do a Google search on him you won't find much, and this seems to be deliberate.

Steinberg was the founder and first editor in chief of *The Journal of Lipid Research* (a publication vehicle for supporters of the *diet heart hypothesis*).

Steinberg was Chairman of the Council on Arteriosclerosis of the American Heart Association and from here recommend treating high cholesterol as early as 1969.

Steinberg was co-chair of the Lipid Research Clinics Coronary Primary Prevention Trial (LRC-CPPT). This trial was led by the National Institutes of Health (NIH), costing $150 million of taxpayer cash.

In January 1984 the results of this trial were published and claimed that evidence was now clear that statins were effective – despite the fact that absolute differentials were negligible in groups observed.

Steinberg was Merck's scientific advisor when lovastatin was approved in record time in 1984. (A bit of a conflict of interest then!)

Steinberg was the first speaker at the FDA advisory committee meeting on statins, held at the NIH, in February 1987.

I hope this small example makes it clear how individuals can influence both government guidelines, medical policy and public opinion on a medication, whilst being paid as a consultant by companies that manufacture these medications.

If you have been prescribed statins, and you are unsure about whether you should take them, then do some research.

One of the best resources that summarises the results of clinical trials and epidemiological studies on statin use is a book by David Evans called ***Statins Toxic Side Effects - Evidence From 500 Scientific Papers***.

I recommend this book if you really want to dig into the facts about statins. It provides the details of the research and summarises the data.

Why every doctor hasn't seen a copy I have no idea!

In chapter 3 of the book, for example, entitled ***"It's official: Statins increase the risk of diabetes"*** there are notes from Evans, and references on 25 papers that demonstrate the conclusion that statins, do in fact, increase the risk of diabetes.

But what do you think is the first thing your doctor will do if you are diagnosed with type 2 diabetes?

He will prescribe you a statin!

I don't think you should take a decision about whether to take statins lightly.

I am **NOT** going to tell you **NOT** to take a statin. That is your decision.

But please, please, please....do not be one of the people that just blindly accepts a medication that has been shown to do so much harm, and whose efficacy is non-existent but for a tiny proportion of sufferers. Be inquisitive, and challenge your doctor. Knowledge is power!

Part 3: Who Is At Risk?

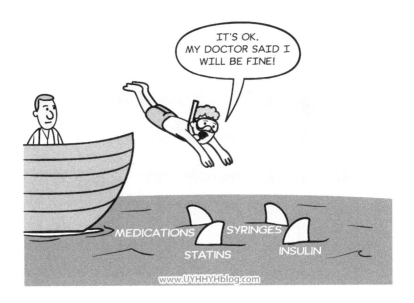

Nan's Chapter Summary: *There are some groups of people that are higher-risk for heart disease than others.*

Those that suffer from clinical depression or anxiety have an increased risk of heart disease, because these mental illnesses increase stress hormones in the body that restrict blood flow through the arteries and increase blood pressure.

They also suffer from an increase in hormones that interfere with good management of blood sugar, and reduce the strength of the immune system.

People that suffer from high blood pressure are also at an increased risk of damaging their artery walls, and putting the heart under more strain.

People with type 2 diabetes are at higher risk of heart disease because they are unable to manage their blood sugar properly, and require insulin injections.

Lastly, men are at higher risk for heart disease than women....at least up until women reach menopause, after which they catch-up with men quite quickly. It is believed that oestrogen helps to protect women from heart disease, but after menopause when this hormone is no longer produced as much women's risk increases. By the time they are 65 women and men have the same amount of heart disease risk.

THE ANXIOUS & DEPRESSED

People with anxiety and depression are high-risk for heart disease.

In 2014 the World Health Organisation stated:

"The average lifetime prevalence of depression has been estimated at 14.6% in high-income countries, 11.1% in low-to middle-income countries. Depression will become the second leading cause of disability-adjusted life years lost by the year 2020."

This was a shocking prediction back then, but having volunteered as a listener for Samaritans for 3 years I can attest to the large number of people that suffer with depression, anxiety and other related mental health issues, that struggle to receive support for these debilitating conditions. It would seem they were correct in presuming this issue would get worse.

But it is not just emotional and cognitive health that is challenged through un-resolved mental illness, physical health for those suffering is severely compromised too, and sometimes with devastating consequences.

Those that suffer depression, anxiety and other mental health issues are at a significant increased risk of heart disease, the biggest killer on the planet.

In 2014, an American Heart Association statement listed depression as a risk factor for a poor prognosis after a heart attack or unstable angina (chest pain at rest due to reduced blood flow to the heart).

One study found that the risk of death in heart attack survivors with depression was three times that of those without depression.

A 2014 Meta-analysis [1] of 30 studies & 40 independent reports that met the inclusion criteria, were analysed. These covered 893,850 participants between 1993 & 2014.

This meta-analysis concluded:

"*Depression is independently associated with a significantly increased risk of Coronary Heart Disease and Myocardial Infarction.*"

This revelation crystallises how important it is to ensure that sufferers seek help to resolve their mental health issues as soon as they can, to avoid them becoming life-threatening physical complications.

One of the reasons that mental illness increases heart disease risk is because it creates a chronic elevation of cortisol.

Cortisol is an important hormone produced by the adrenal glands. It is secreted by the body in response to stress and is one of the hormones involved in the 'fight-or-flight' response.

Cortisol plays an important role in everything from how the body uses glucose, to the regulation of blood pressure and the functioning of a healthy immune system.

Cortisol has many benefits, when administered in small doses periodically when needed by the body. It primes you for physical and emotional challenges, facilitates bursts of energy and can provide surges of immune activity when you're confronted with infectious diseases, or an impending physical threat.

All good here, so what's the issue?

---

[1] https://bmcpsychiatry.biomedcentral.com/articles/10.1186/s12888-014-0371-z

When you're exposed to continuous or prolonged stress, which results in chronic over-production of cortisol, you will start to experience negative side effects.

Chronically elevated levels of cortisol throughout the day will increase blood glucose (which in turn elevates insulin chronically) which will in-turn increase fat storage, elevate blood-pressure, suppress your immune system and reduce your ability to fight infections.

Clearly it is a very bad thing to put yourself through chronic stress continually, throughout the day.

If you are wondering what the stressors are that increase cortisol, here are a few.

Feeling anxious or depressed will increase cortisol, which will (frustratingly) make you feel more anxious and depressed, creating a vicious cycle.

Poor sleep, road-rage, fear, poor relationships, a job you hate, being stuck in traffic, an argument with your boss....pretty much anything that triggers anger, sadness and emotional distress will elevate your cortisol.

All of these things tell your brain to activate the sympathetic nervous system and trigger the same chemical reactions that would have elicited a response to moments of danger, in days gone by. Except these days there is no real danger, just the emotional antagonists of modern life.

And instead of this happening periodically, maybe once a week, as is designed to be the case… in our modern, busy lives we experience these things many times every day.

Our bodies are equipped with natural self-repair mechanisms that fight cancer, prevent infection, repair wounds, and protect us from infectious agents and foreign bodies.

These natural self-repair mechanisms are deactivated when the body is full of stress hormones. This suppresses the immune response, which increases the risk of developing all sorts of diseases, including arthritis, cancer, and auto-immune disorders....and the big one....heart disease.

There was a study performed on a small town called Roseto in the early 1960's.

Roseto, Pennsylvania, was a town of mostly Italian population, and was noted to have a "strikingly low" number of deaths from heart disease. The local diet consisted of copious amounts of animal fat, including prosciutto with fat an inch thick around the rim, and most meals cooked in lard.

The population of Roseto habitually ate large meals and drank a lot of wine, and were generally overweight, but not one of them under 50 died of a heart attack during the years of the survey from 1955 to 1961.

This town became quite well known, and was part of a published study in 1964. There are many reasons why the Roseto population of Italian immigrants were somewhat protected from heart disease, and their diet did not seem to have an adverse affect at all.

One of the notable factors was that the residents had emigrated from a specific region of Italy, they had an incredible community spirit and lots of friends and relatives nearby. They lead sociable lives, and had an integrated supportive community. They mainly worked in one large local employer, which provided stable job security.

It was noted, after much ongoing study, that the residents of Roseto were protected from heart disease to a great extent, despite some poor lifestyle choices, because their stress levels were so low.

Ongoing chronic stress ensures that cortisol, and it's co-conspirators adrenaline and insulin are elevated throughout most of the day, wreaking havoc on our bodies and our brain.

This is why anxiety and depression are a significant risk factor for heart disease.

THE HYPERTENSIVE

People with high blood pressure are high-risk for heart disease.

When it leaves the heart, your blood needs to be forced out through *arteries* at such a rate that it can travel the length of your limbs delivering oxygen and nutrients, and then come back through the *veins* to be re-oxygenated in the lungs before repeating the cycle.

The initial pressure as it leaves your heart via the arteries, as you can imagine, is higher than when it returns through the veins.

Did you know that atherosclerosis ("furring" or plaque build-up) NEVER occurs in veins...despite cholesterol running through all of them.

Why is this?

It has been thought for some time that the reason for this is that because the blood pressure is lower in the veins on the way back to the heart (3-8mmHg) than when being forced out by the heart through the arteries (8-20 mmHg) less damage is inflicted on the vein walls.

Anybody who has seen what a jet-wash can do to will attest to the abrasive power of water pressure, so it is unsurprising that a higher force of blood pushed through arteries will damage them, but not veins.

Blood pressure that is elevated for prolonged periods above the requirements for reasonable blood flow, can cause damage to your endothelial walls, the thin layer, once cell thick, that lines the inside of your arteries.

Once this damage occurs, your body sends its repair mechanism (LDL) to the damaged area. Small LDL particles can become lodged in damaged artery walls, and problems may ensue if these LDL particles have been exposed to oxidation, through inflammatory conditions.

This can start a cascade of events that ultimately leads to plaque formation, and eventually a reduced artery "aperture", which may become blocked through a blood clot or unstable plaque rupture.

So keeping your blood pressure at a healthy level is a pretty important factor in preventing this unfortunate series of events from starting in the first place.

But before you go into a wild panic to reduce your blood pressure by all means necessary to the lowest level possible, you need to understand that blood pressure that is too low also has a number of issues, so understanding what is "normal" is quite important.

When measuring systolic and diastolic blood pressure we are told that the goal is 120/80 for optimum health, but this is a bit of an idealistic target.

The reality is that as we age our blood pressure naturally increases even though it remains in a healthy range for our age, and is not damaging.

A reasonable view of "normal" blood pressure has, for a long time, been thought to be a systolic number of (100 + age) over a diastolic number of 80 if under 40 years of age (85 if you are over 40 years of age).

Recently, however, advice has changed again, and advice has changed to limit systolic blood pressure to 140 or under.[2]

Remember though, we are all different, so there is a range of normal either side of these numbers that may be *your* normal.

I am 53, so I have been reasonably happy with blood pressure of 153/85 (100 plus my age over 85 as I am over 40) or under, but recent studies seem to suggest that above 140 as a systolic measurement, regardless of age is the point at which blood pressure should start to be managed down.[3]

If I started to see a regular pattern of 10% above this level, I would take action to reduce my blood pressure, but I wouldn't panic if my blood pressure was 140/85 for example, and I certainly wouldn't go onto blood pressure medication (although many doctors would prescribe it at this level).

Blood pressure medications tend to have a very high propensity for some very unpleasant and damaging side effects, and they also have pretty low efficacy for results.

In a study titled ***Drug Side Effect Symptoms And Adherence To Antihypertensive Medication*** from 2016, the study researchers concluded that;

"Eighty-five percent of the participants experienced side effects."

These side effects included:

"Anticholinergic (dry mouth, blurry vision, and vision problems); Gastrointestinal (heartburn and vomiting); Genitourinary (increased urination, getting up often during the night to empty bladder, problems in gaining an erection, and decreased interest in sex); Cardio-pulmonary (cough, swelling of feet or ankles, and shortness of breath); Functional impairment (fatigue, general weakness, lethargy, and

---

[3]   https://pubmed.ncbi.nlm.nih.gov/12748199/

tiredness); Neuro-psychiatric and cognitive (numbness or tingling of hand, insomnia, mood swings, feeling depressed, and difficult remembering things); Miscellaneous (itching, weight gain, and muscle cramp)."

For example, Lotensin (a well known blood pressure medication) has side effects that in one trial [4] were recorded thus:

"The most frequently reported adverse events were peripheral oedema (circa 12% of the test group), headache, cough, upper respiratory-tract infection, fatigue, nasopharyngitis (swelling of the nasal passages and the back of the throat), diarrhoea, dizziness and muscle cramp."

Peripheral oedema is swelling of your lower legs or hands.

All of these side effects were experienced in order to gain a 10% to 15% reduction in blood pressure from using Lotensin, in a group of subjects with really high blood pressure.

This level of reduction is very commonly seen within a few weeks of lifestyle and therapeutic changes without any medication at all, and with no side effects.

In a trial called the MRC Trial,[5] of the 17,354 patients with mild hypertension (over 160/110…yep that's "mild") half were treated with blood pressure medication and half with a placebo.

After 9 years no difference was noted in cardio-vascular mortality between the groups.

---

[4]   https://www.nature.com/articles/jhh200980

[5]   https://pubmed.ncbi.nlm.nih.gov/2861880/

"Treatment made no difference to the overall rates of coronary events." the study organisers concluded.

You may believe that salt intake can increase your blood pressure, and that reducing salt will improve it. This idea came about as it was concluded that salt attracts water, and therefore must increase water volume, therefore increasing blood volume and applying more pressure to your arteries and veins.

This seems logical, but is overly simplistic, and is not where we should focus attention to lower high blood pressure.

As Ben Bikman states in *Why We Get Sick;*

"For decades medical practitioners have been recommending we eat less salt. The thought is that getting too little salt is better than the risk of consuming too much. Unfortunately, this is simply incorrect."

Apparently when salt is restricted in our diet our liver initiates a process to extract as much as possible back from our urine into the blood. Aldosterone assists in this job, whilst at the same time antagonising insulin, and contributing to insulin resistance.

Additionally, Dr Malcom Kendrick notes that reducing salt *"Fires-up RAAS"* (Renin-Angiotensin System), which in-turn activates the sympathetic nervous system…in other words the stress response in the body, which constricts blood vessels and decreases nitric oxide synthesis….this process he describes as;

"Almost perfectly designed to increase risk of cardiovascular disease!"

Aldosterone secreted from the adrenal glands, regulates salt and water and it signals our kidneys to hold on to salt.

Insulin increases aldosterone and, therefore, elevated insulin can lead to raised blood pressure. Insulin becomes elevated when we are insulin resistant or when we eat sugar or high glycemic foods.

As Ben Bikman concludes in **Why We Get Sick;**

"We're coming to understand that insulin resistance and high insulin levels directly cause high blood pressure."

Ivor Cummins states in his podcast **The Fat Emperor;**

"Hypertension is reverseable and is insulin resistance until proven otherwise."

So one effective way to decrease our blood pressure is to adopt a low glycemic diet (like the ketogenic diet that we will cover later in the book), or to fast periodically (we will cover this too).

Another factor in elevated blood pressure is stress. Stress hormones actually stiffen artery walls, increasing our blood pressure ready for a surge of dynamic "fight-or-flight" activity.

Imagine your artery as a hosepipe, turn on the tap a little, and the water flows out. If you narrow the aperture through which the water passes, the pressure becomes greater and the water travels out more quickly. The stiffer and narrower the hosepipe the higher the water pressure becomes.

Chronic stress (ie stress occurring too frequently) will maintain stiff artery walls for longer, creating high blood pressure.

This is why the best advice to reduce blood pressure is actually to manage insulin and stress hormones, not to focus on consumption of salt.

There are many things that can help reduce blood pressure, such as regular moderate exercise and even heat treatments like sauna taken regularly.

In an article published in the ***American Journal of Hypertension*** [6] the findings of a Finnish study of 1,621 middle-aged men with hypertension were noted. The ***Kuopio Ischaemic Heart Disease Risk Factor Study (KIHD)***, monitored the men over a 22 year period, and divided them into groups that engaged in varying frequencies of sauna use.

The researchers concluded that;

"The risk of hypertension was 24% decreased among men with a sauna frequency of 2-3 times a week, and 46% lowered among men who had a sauna 4-7 times a week."

Regular sauna use for circa 20 minutes at a time, at least 2 to 3 times per week seems to have some great health benefits.

In the scholarly article ***Is sauna bathing protective of sudden cardiac death? A review of the evidence*** the authors concluded;

"Plausible pathways underlying the protective effect of sauna bathing on sudden cardiac death may be linked to the impact on cardiovascular function via reduced arterial stiffness, decreases in inflammation and oxidative stress, stabilisation of the autonomic nervous system, beneficial changes in circulating lipid profiles and other CVD risk markers, and lowering of systemic blood pressure."

---

[6]   https://www.sciencedaily.com/releases/2017/09/170929093346.htm

THE DIABETIC (& PRE-DIABETIC)

People with diabetes and pre-diabetes (insulin resistance, metabolic syndrome) are high-risk for heart disease.

Type 2 diabetes is a serious disease that can be avoided through physical activity, diet, and lifestyle yet it is one of the leading causes of death in the western world and is a massive cost to health services globally.

Pre-diabetes is the path leading to type 2 diabetes, where our body's are starting to show the metabolic dysregulation that if left un-checked will inevitably lead us there.

Metabolic syndrome and insulin resistance are terms used to describe those with type 2 diabetes and pre-diabetes, hose on a trajectory to develop full type 2 diabetes unless they modify their lifestyles.

Pre-diabetes is often specifically used to describe somebody that is expected to become type 2 diabetic within a 5 year period….so when a medical refers to us in these terms we don't have much time left to act.

As of 2015, 30.3 million Americans – 9.4% of the U.S. population – had diabetes. Another 84.1 million had pre-diabetes.

Dr Mark Hyman recently stated that it is estimated that 88% of Americans are pre-diabetic or insulin resistant.

People with diabetes are at increased risk of serious health complications including:

- vision loss

- heart disease

- stroke

- kidney failure

- impotence

- dementia

- depression

- amputation of toes, feet, or legs

The costs:

- $327 billion: Total cost of diagnosed diabetes in the United States in 2017
- $237 billion for direct medical costs and $90 billion for reduced productivity

After adjusting for population age and sex differences, average medical expenditure among people with diagnosed diabetes were 2.3 times higher than non diabeteics.

CDC Director Brenda Fitzgerald, M.D. said in 2015;

"More than a third of U.S. adults have pre-diabetes, and the majority don't know it. Now, more than ever, we must step up our efforts to reduce the burden of this serious disease."

Diabetes was once thought irreversible, but now it is clear from research that type 2 diabetes can be avoided, and even reversed through diet and lifestyle adaptations.

A diet that minimises sugar and maintains a low glycemic load, is shown to have a positive impact on reducing metabolic syndrome, preventing type 2 diabetes and reversing it.

One style of diet that encapsulates this ethos is the ketogenic diet.

These diets prioritise fats, protein and non-starchy foods over starchy vegetables, grains and carbohydrates.

175

The effect of this type of eating plan is to reduce or eradicate the elevated insulin that creates metabolic syndrome and leads to insulin resistance and type 2 diabetes.

James Muecke, A leading eye specialist in Australia who treats diabetes induced blindness regularly and Australian of the Year 2020, has this to say on the subject.

Speaking about the food pyramid we use in the western world prioritising bread, grains and cereals he said;

"It is time to start dealing with the toxic impact of sugar. I want Australians to be aware our dietary guidelines are flawed, and the authors conflicted by industry."

He went on to say.

"I want Australians to know they can eat eggs, full-fat dairy and red meat without fearing for their lives or eternal damnation."

What will seem strange when you look at the public organisational guidelines for treatment of diabetes, is that despite all the science (and the obvious logic) supporting the reduction of insulin (through a reduction in blood-sugar) as the primary treatment for diabetes, the public health institutions have been resistant to recommend these interventions.

The hypocrisy of the American Diabetes Association is frustrating and very clear.

For instance it calls it a "myth" that sugar causes type 2 diabetes because they claim it is caused by "genetics and lifestyle factors" that make us fat. They then proceed to recommend that we all avoid sugar sweetened beverages to prevent diabetes.

This same organisation then accepts the role of fat accumulation in the liver as quite possibly a causal factor in the development of insulin resistance, diabetes and obesity......but ignores the evidence that implicate sugar as the cause of hepatic (liver) fat accumulation.

I discussed the political and financial interests of the American Heart Association, big Pharma, big Agriculture and the various sugar industry organisations.

As a consequence of these commercial interests, even in the face of the scientific facts, the correct lifestyle changes are not readily promoted through some of the very bodies that are tasked with supporting our good health.

Insulin resistance/type 2 diabetes is something that we should pay particular attention to because:

- We can create it through poor lifestyle choices

- We can reverse it through good lifestyle choices

- Once we create this in ourselves, this susceptibility can be passed on to our unborn children!

So how do we become insulin resistant?

Dr Benjamin Bikman authored the awesome book *Why We Get Sick* which explains everything we would ever need to know, and more, about the causes and effects of insulin resistance.

In a podcast [7] hosted by leading bodybuilder Ben Pakulski, Dr Bikman explained that too much of a substance in the body may cause a resistance to that substance, and went on to say that;

"If someone is living their life, chronically bumping-up their insulin, maybe every 2-3 hours because they are told to eat high carbohydrate snacks and keep their energy high,

---

then they are living every waking moment in a state of elevated insulin."

To put this into context, the podcast is aimed at fitness athletes and bodybuilders, a community that generally advocates eating 6 meals a day as the healthiest way to ensure that energy levels and nutrients are always present to feed muscles recovering from exercise. It is not uncommon for this group of people to eat every 3 hours.

Dr Bikman was highlighting the challenges that come with this kind of consistent and regular eating pattern.

But how different is this really from the eating patterns of many of us?

It is not uncommon for many people to have 3 meals a day and to snack in-between meals, which will have a similar effect.

Breakfast, then a snack during the day (or a tea or coffee with sugar in it…same effect), then lunch, and a snack on the way home from work in the car, then dinner, then a beer or two in the evening.

This creates a constantly elevated state of insulin in the blood.

He continues;

"If you are eating a carbohydrate-rich meal, your insulin will be up, depending on the person, for anywhere between 2-4 hours."

He goes on to explain that by the time we finally relieve our bodies of circulating insulin, when sleeping, we are soon waking-up to start the whole cycle again the next day.

In Dr Bikmans book he provides some helpful tips on how, most without the need for a blood test, we can estimate whether we are one of the roughly 80% of adults in the western world that is insulin resistant.

Look at the list below:

- More fat on your belly

- High blood pressure

- Family history of heart disease

- Retain water easily

- Patches of darker skin, or skin tags, on neck or armpits

- High blood triglycerides (fat circulating in the blood....this can be seen in. A standard blood test)

- Family member with diabetes

- PCOS (polycystic ovary syndrome)

- Erectile dysfunction

Dr Bikman suggests that if one of these items applies to you, then it is possible that you are insulin resistant.

If two or more apply to you, then you are certain to be insulin resistant

GENETICS AGAIN

Genetics loads the gun! Lifestyle pulls the trigger!

People with genetic pre-dispositions are high-risk for heart disease.

Genetic factors are a significant issue for heart health in a couple of ways, even aside for the genetic levels of cholesterol that I covered in an earlier chapter on FH.

We may unfortunately inherit a gene expression from our parents that produces too much of a problematic element like my genetically high LP(a) or maybe a clotting factor like fibrinogen for example, and this will inevitably make some of us more likely to develop atherosclerosis or experience a heart attack, or develop it faster, than those of us with more moderate gene expression.

Whilst this is unfortunate, it is hardly something our parents could be expected to know, and even if they did, there is often little they can do to prevent genes being passed to their children.

Some other genetic factors though, are in fact more a result of our parents lifestyles than their genetics. These are ones that we might do well to manage, both for our own health and to prevent our children from inheriting them and passing them on to their children.

Insulin resistance and type 2 diabetes are brought-on by lifestyle, but seemingly can also be passed-on to children from parents.

A 2009 study [8] had the purpose of determining whether foetuses of obese women have increased obesity, insulin resistance, and markers of inflammation, supporting the concept of foetal programming.

---

[8]   https://care.diabetesjournals.org/content/32/6/1076

The study concluded that;

"Data suggest that maternal obesity creates a significant risk for the next generations with metabolic compromise already apparent at birth."

Gary Taubes in *The Case Against Sugar* writes;

"45% of the children of diabetic mothers become diabetic themselves by the time they're in their mid 20s."

This is more than 30 times the rate of diabetes seen in children of mothers who remained healthy.

Having high blood sugar or being insulin resistance and glucose intolerant while pregnant, is passed from mother to child in the womb... this is known as "metabolic imprinting".

This should be a significant wake-up call to us all.

It is common these days for women that previously smoke cigarettes, to decide to give-up smoking when they are pregnant, or adapt their diets, knowing that while they are pregnant the things they consume may affect their unborn child.

It is a bigger responsibility still to think that we can pre-determine an increase in chronic illness, or heart disease risk for our children, from *our* lifestyles choices long before pregnancy though.

Ethnicity seems to also play a factor in the genetics.

It has long been known that certain ethnicities have a greater predisposition to diabetes for example.

A study [9] examining the different prevalence of diabetes on ethnic groups in the United States concluded there was;

"A drastic difference in insulin sensitivity among the different ethnic groups."

They had studied the differences between Hispanic, Asian, African and "Caucasian" Americans.

Knowing your genetic risk profile is an important factor, and can help to target treatment and prevention protocols. This is covered later in testing, so you can understand what genetic factors may play a part in your risk.

Almost all genetic factors can be mitigated to some degree by the right lifestyle interventions.

A genetically loaded gun can't hurt you, if you don't pull the trigger!

---

[9]   https://care.diabetesjournals.org/content/23/9/1353

MEN

Men are at high-risk for heart disease.

That's right, women and men have quite different profiles for heart disease.

And for a change, it is men that are the victims of this particular form of health sexism.

Men are far more likely to have heart attacks than women, well at least up until about the age of 65, after which the risks are broadly the same for men and women.

After menopause, the protection women have over men in athero-sclerotic progression seems to disappear.

Largely due to the protective properties of oestrogen, cardiovascular disease develops (or rather is statistically evident) 7 to 10 years later in women than in men, but it is worth noting that it is *still the major cause of death in women over the age of 65 years old.*

To some doctors, the risk of heart disease in women may sometimes be underestimated, due to the understanding that women are 'protected' against cardiovascular disease by oestrogen, but of course after the menopause the protection is no longer provided.

There is no room for complacency regarding risk factors, however.

Damage may still be initiated to the cardiovascular system of women before menopause. Some studies [10] have shown that whilst arterial damage can still be created, the effects of this damage may be delayed until after menopause, when they will have a greater effect.

---

[10]   https://www.ncbi.nlm.nih.gov/pmc/articles/PMC3018605/

For these reasons, women should not take the view that oestrogen is some kind of free-pass to avoid heart disease......it may just take a little longer before the effects take their toll.

Oestrogens have a regulating effect on several key heart-health factors, such as fats in the blood, inflammatory markers and blood-clotting, so it seems logical that women have more positive outcomes at the time of their lives when oestrogen is present.

In the Women's Ischemia Syndrome Evaluation (WISE) study [11] it was shown that young women with an oestrogen deficiency have a more than sevenfold increase in coronary artery risk than women without the deficiency.

---

[11]

https://www.ahajournals.org/doi/10.1161/CIRCOUTCOMES.116
.003863

WHO SHOULD GET TESTED & WHY?

Nan's Chapter Summary: *There are some tests which can help to show if a person is likely to be susceptible to heart disease, or if it has already started.*

The best test to establish any existing blockage in the arteries is a scan that can measure the calcium that is lodged in your artery walls. This is called a calcium CT scan.

Any man over 40 or woman over 50 that is concerned about whether they are at risk should start by taking this test.

Many other tests are available that can establish if there are any genetic factors that you have inherited that put you at high-risk. Levels of cholesterol are not good predictors of heart health, and are not of much use.

There are some tests that can show if your body is managing to maintain a good hormone balance. There are also tests that show if you have genetics that might be problematic, and there are also some tests that show if your body is experiencing high levels of internal inflammation.

All of these tests can be used to establish if you might need to adjust your lifestyle, or diet to reduce your heart disease risk.

Now that we have a clearer understanding of what actually causes heart disease, we can be clearer about which tests will provide the best indicators for risk.

One of the biggest challenges with the misguided beliefs that pervade today relating to saturated fat and cholesterol as the main causes for heart disease, is that they have led to standard blood tests which look at the wrong measurements to ascertain risk.

Because of this challenge, it is highly likely that in order to ascertain your true risk you will need a series of tests that will not be available from your GP.

Testing for risk needs to be appropriately deep, to avoid misdiagnosis, particularly if you are somebody that doesn't fit the "standard risk-profile" that doctors are trained to look for.

As a rule of thumb, I would suggest the following 3 groups of people should undergo tests for heart disease risk regardless of any other factors; men over 40, women over 50 & any adult over the age of 30 with a family history of early heart disease.

MEN OVER 40

If you are a man over 40, but are generally healthy, what can I do to convince you that you should be tested for heart disease risk?

In fact, if you fit that profile, you probably aren't even reading this book.

And why would you?

3 years ago I wouldn't have read this book either. I was the last person that was going to experience a heart attack, as a relatively fit 49 year-old man.

If you are a seemingly healthy man in your forties or fifties, you probably don't feel remotely vulnerable to heart disease either, and if that is the case, why waste time reading a book on the subject, when you could be out with friends, or sitting down to an evening watching Netflix?

I am with you 100%.

Except, that for one reason or another, it is likely that a good percentage of you are creating an environment to develop heart disease already, and it may well be quite advanced.

Men are at higher-risk from heart disease than women, before the age of 65.

According to a 2016 study in Norway,[12] which included nearly 34,000 people;

---

[12]   https://www.health.harvard.edu/heart-health/throughout-life-heart-attacks-are-twice-as-common-in-men-than-women

"Researchers found that throughout life, men were about twice as likely as women to have a heart attack. That higher risk persisted even after they accounted for traditional risk factors for heart disease, including high cholesterol, high blood pressure, diabetes, body mass index, and physical activity."

Although female sex hormones play a role in protecting women from atherosclerosis somewhat, the researchers in this particular study think there is more to it than that as they noticed that;

"The risk of heart attack changed only slightly as women transitioned through menopause, making it unlikely that female hormone levels explain these findings."

There are many factors, as well as the seemingly protective effects of oestrogen, that may determine the increased risk of heart disease for men.

For example, men don't talk!

Whether it is money worries, a health issue, stress at work, relationship problems, men don't tend to talk about their problems with other men, or with their partners or families or friends in many cases.

"Men do have emotionally meaningful friendships, which are important to them, however they do not tend to talk to their friends about emotional issues on a regular basis." states one Samaritans study from 2016.

Samaritans offers listening support for this in times of need, and their vision is that fewer people die by suicide, as a result of having somebody to talk to.

Every year, Samaritans volunteers spend over one million hours answering calls for help via their 24-hour service.

A significant proportion of the calls and texts received are from women, and they generally called to talk through their challenges long before they become so overwhelming that suicide is contemplated.

Men, however, call far less frequently, and when they do they are often already feeling quite hopeless and resigned, and often confirm that they have kept their problems a secret from friends, family and colleagues.

Statistics from Samaritans for 2017 show that 75% of suicides in the UK are committed by men, even though this is the lowest suicide rate for men in 30 years.

14 in every 100,000 men and 4.6 in every 100,000 women committed suicide in England in 2017.

The highest rate for suicide in the UK is in men between the ages of 45 and 49.

The UK Office for National Statistics [13] issued figures relating to suicides and stated;

"Three-quarters of registered deaths in 2018 were among men (4,903 deaths), which has been the case since the mid-1990s".

If you are wondering what this has to do with heart disease in men, then this quote from Malcolm Kendrick in A Statin Nation provides a clue;

---

[13]

https://www.ons.gov.uk/peoplepopulationandcommunity/birthsde athsandmarriages/deaths/bulletins/suicidesintheunitedkingdom/2018 registrations

"Researchers found that people who suffer from significant money worries are 13 times more likely to suffer a heart attack".

If mental health issues like financial pressures, anxiety, depression and loneliness are risk-factors for heart disease, then men that don't seek help to resolve their problems are more likely to increase their heart disease risk.

In a 2019 survey by Samaritans they found one in four men (25%) in Ireland who had suicidal thoughts in the previous 12 months did not reach out for help due to feeling like they had no one to trust, with 37% feeling like a burden.

The survey found that some of the main reasons why men find life tough and struggle include job loss/employment issues (38%), relationship or family problems (38%), and debt or financial worries (37%).

They discovered six out of ten (57%) men who experienced a life crisis in the previous year did not look for help as they preferred to try and solve their problems themselves. 36% of men said they felt "alone".

"Our survey results found that although 76% of men say it's okay to admit you're not feeling okay, many still avoid speaking out when they're finding life tough." the organisation concluded.

Similarly, when men are less likely to see a doctor when they have an infection or inflammatory condition, again they will increase their risk for heart disease.

In a 2008/9 study by Men's Health Forum[14] it was shown that men are much less likely than women to visit a GP.

They found;

"In persons aged 20-40 women attended a general practice twice as often."

They also noted that;

"men are less likely than women to acknowledge illness or to seek help when sick" and are *"twice as likely to have inadequate health literacy."*

These, along with gender specific hormones, are just a few of many factors which contribute to mens greater risk of heart disease compared to women (pre menopause).

The fact remains that there is a significantly greater risk of heart disease for men under 65 than women under 65.

---

[14]   https://www.menshealthforum.org.uk/key-data-understanding-health-and-access-services

WOMEN OVER 50

Why women over 50?

Cardiovascular disease is the leading cause of death for both women and men (1 in every 3 deaths in the United States).

However, CVD in women rarely occurs[15] before the 6th decade of life.

It has been suggested that reduction of female sex hormones, specifically oestrogen, in menopause is related to increased CVD risk in women as they age.

As mentioned before, men over 40 start to show the tell-tale signs of heart disease.

Women, however, are somewhat protected from heart disease before the menopause, and by implication by female sex hormones, particularly oestrogen.

Oestrogen's "known" effects on the cardiovascular system include a mix of positive and negative:

- Increases HDL cholesterol

- Decreases LDL cholesterol

- Promotes blood clot formation, but also causes some changes that have the opposite effect

- Relaxes, smooths and dilates blood vessels so blood flow increases

---

[15]   https://pubmed.ncbi.nlm.nih.gov/8602000/

- Soaks up free radicals, naturally occurring particles in the blood that can damage the arteries and other tissues.

Oestrogen probably affects the cardiovascular system in other ways that are as yet undiscovered.

Research continues to give scientists and physicians more information – and raise more questions about this important heart-health hormone.

Heart disease remains the number one killer among women over age 65, and although women develop heart disease 10 years later than men, by age 65, their risk is equal to that of men.

For this reason, I advise that women of 50 would probably be at a similar stage of risk to men of 40, and I would advise that women from the age of 50 should test for heart disease risk.

A 2010 article[16] entitled *Gender Differences In Coronary Heart Disease* states that;

"Cardiovascular disease develops 7 to 10 years later in women than in men and is still the major cause of death in women".

"Women with acute coronary syndrome are generally older with more clustering of risk factors that may contribute to their higher risk of mortality."

---

[16]   https://www.ncbi.nlm.nih.gov/pmc/articles/PMC3018605/

ANY ADULT WITH FAMILY HISTORY

Regardless of your sex, if you have family history of heart disease in early adulthood, then you should be tested for heart disease risk.

Despite the fact that heart disease is a factor of hormone imbalance and inflammation, it can be accelerated and exacerbated by genetics.

This is something I have discovered in my particular case.

Whilst I was considered extremely low-risk from a blood profile test and lifestyle questionnaire, and had no traditional signs of heart disease risk, I suffered a near fatal heart attack, and if my GP had any idea of what to look for to judge my risk, it would have been very clear that I was a high-risk patient.

I had high LP(a).

Not just a bit high, but 300% of the upper level of normal.

High LP(a) essentially makes you a heart attack victim waiting to happen.

My cardiologist (in my post-operative briefing) said to me "In a line-up of 100 people, you are about the last person I would have guessed would be at risk!"

He, like my GP, was mistaken in assuming my risk was low, by only looking at my:

- Total cholesterol (normal to low)

- Triglycerides (very low)

- Lifestyle (non-smoker, fit)

- Weight and BMI (normal)

- Blood pressure (normal)

These were the only metrics that were assessed by my GP before my heart attack, and worryingly, neither GP or the cardiologist saw any benefit in testing further afterwards to find the cause of my CVD.

As far as the medical establishment was concerned, the cause of my CVD was of no relevance.

I can only assume that this is because the treatment protocol was going to be the same regardless of what had caused my CVD, namely:

- Lower cholesterol through prescription of *Atorvastatin* (despite the fact that this does NOT decrease CVD risk)

- Lower blood pressure through prescription of *Ramipril* (despite the fact that blood pressure was in the normal range)

- Prevent blood clotting through prescription of *Clopidogrel* (used as a double-whammy with the Aspirin)

- Prevent blood clotting through prescription of *Aspirin*

- Manage some of the stomach issues created by all of the prescriptions above, through prescription of *Ranitidine*

- Exercise at least 10,000 steps a day (I was already doing more than this)

- Eat less cholesterol (despite the fact that cholesterol is genetically determined and eating less makes no difference to levels in the blood, and the fact that my cholesterol was normal and healthy)

I had to go and find a test for "everything" and work out for myself what the meaning of "it must just be genetic" actually meant in my case.

Why is this important?

Well for one thing, I now know that I have to be very, very careful to avoid the things that cause inflammation as my body is likely to react less positively than most other people, due to my high LP(a) count and particle size.

I also now know that a particular vitamin and diet supplementation strategy can reduce my LP(a) slightly, and can reduce the adhesive qualities of the LP(a) that is circulating.

I can also repair my arterial walls through supplementing to improve my collagen production.

None of the standard NHS medical interventions or advice would have achieved any of these improvements, and I would not have lowered my specific risk for heart disease.

An additional concern with the comment that I received from my cardiologist and doctor of "it must just be genetic", is that I may have passed my risk factors on to my children, and my siblings may well be susceptible to heart disease too if they have the same genetic profile.

N.B. As I write this, my brother, 2 years younger than me (at 50 now) has just been advised that he needs a triple bypass! He had no idea he was at high risk either! He weighs 11 stone and doesn't have high blood pressure or diabetes, although he is a smoker.

We have discovered a somewhat tenuous link to heart disease in two men on my mothers side of the family.

Ironically, we thought we were so much healthier than my grandparents generation growing-up on a diet of skimmed milk, cereal, bread and margarine, with chicken and no red meat.

How wrong we were!

Any adult with a family history should test for the likely genetic factors for heart disease.

I have listed a selection of the most valuable tests in the next section, so you can understand if you have a genetic risk factor or a lifestyle risk factor that you should work to mitigate.

WHAT PREDICTS HEART DISEASE RISK & WHAT DOESN'T!

By now you will realise that I am an advocate of maintaining a healthy cholesterol level (that means keeping it high enough to be a health asset), and that I am firmly of the belief that it is not a predictor of heart disease, based on statistical evidence and all unbiased reliable data.

By now you will realise that This doesn't mean that there aren't measurements that can reliably predict heart disease risk though.

THE MEASUREMENTS THAT DON'T MATTER

Nan's Chapter Summary: Testing your cholesterol levels will provide some information on the levels of HDL relative to LDL, and it will tell you an HDL number that you can add to a ratio with triglycerides in your blood, but your cholesterol level doesn't tell you much about your heart disease risk.

LDL Cholesterol & Total Cholesterol (unless they are too low)

There really is very little that you can learn about your heart disease risk by looking at total cholesterol or LDL in isolation or HDL in isolation.

It is actually quite daft that doctors continue to spout these numbers, and test almost exclusively for these two lipoproteins.

You should not feel safe with low LDL and you should not feel safe with high HDL.

You should not feel worried with high LDL.

You may feel a little concerned with low HDL…but that can be elevated with the right diet.

Aside from these with a genetic pre-disposition to abnormally high cholesterol (FH discussed earlier) the only real concern that I would have about LDL and total cholesterol is if it is too low.

This has consistently been linked to increased mortality, shorter life expectancy and a myriad of life-limiting conditions which one would want to avoid.

Those over 60 with high cholesterol have less infections and disease and have a greater life expectancy than those with normal or low LDL, thanks to the immune-supporting properties of LDL.

THE MEASUREMENTS THAT MATTER

Nan's Chapter Summary: *These are the measurements that you might consider checking when assessing for heart disease risk.*

Many of these measurements are not available through a standard GP blood test, and may not even be available through the NHS at all, so you may need to arrange a private test.

There are some companies that package-up a panel that include most or all of these though, and links are provided at the back of the book.

If you have already experienced heart disease, or feel you are at medium to high risk, or if you are a man over 40 and a woman over 50, I would strongly suggest that you look to test for all of the below.

Calcium CT Scan

Nan's Chapter Summary: *A calcium CT scan checks for calcium in your artery walls. It can tell you specifically if you already have blocked, or partially blocked arteries.*

A calcium CT scan is the "gold standard" of tests to show whether calcification has started to form on your arteries.

The result of the test is usually given as a number called an Agatston score.

The score reflects the total area of calcium deposits and the density of the calcium.

A score of zero means no calcium is seen in the heart. It suggests a low chance of developing a heart attack in the future.

When calcium is present, the higher the score, the higher your risk of heart disease.

A score of 100 to 300 means moderate plaque deposits. It is associated with a relatively high risk of heart attack or other heart disease over the next three to five years.

A score greater than 300 is a sign of very high to severe disease and heart attack risk.

Many hospitals in the UK will provide a Calcium CT Scan, often known as a CAC scan.

I firmly believe that if you are a man over 40 and a woman over 50 this should be a standard scan performed every 5 years as part of a heart-health screening programme.

It is a real-time picture of the extent of any calcification that has already formed.

If you get a zero, you are "golden", regardless of all other risk factors, as you will know that you do NOT currently have any atherosclerosis.

If you have *no risk factors, but you score over 300 you have a very high risk of a heart attack*, but you have a chance to take action and understand the root causes.

If this was a standard test, there would be no such thing as a surprise heart attack, and hundreds of thousands of lives would be saved every year.

If you would like to find the nearest scan centre to you, in the UK and Ireland then go to www.ihda.ie which is the website for Irish Heart Disease Awareness, where they provide all the details of where this test can be performed.

It is not cheap to have the test, but if you are a man over 40 or a woman over 50, please consider booking yourself in for a test, if for no other reason than to put your mind at rest.

Triglycerides to HDL

Nan's Chapter Summary: The TG/HDL ratio is available from your GP and can highlight a risk if it is high. This shows the level of triglycerides in the blood and your body's ability to remove them. It can indicate that you may have a problem managing blood sugar.

Ivor Cummins hosts The Fat Emperor podcast.

He is an ex engineer, who now spends his time interviewing experts from around the world....scientists and doctors that have un-picked the science and the data behind chronic diseases such as cardiovascular disease.

When asked which are the tests that he considers most valuable Ivor suggested initially total cholesterol to HDL ratio and triglyceride to HDL ratio....but not because they provide any meaningful information on cholesterol, but instead because they act as a useful proxy to inform the metabolic health of an individual, in the absence of being able to measure the relationship between glucose and insulin easily.

"I would overwhelmingly focus on the ratios of total cholesterol to HDL and triglyceride to HDL as the most valuable markers from a standard cholesterol panel. Doctors just look at total and LDL and they don't realise that these ratios are a pretty good proxy for insulin resistance. The best thing from the cholesterol "panel" is that it mimics or it's a proxy for something else that's not to do with cholesterol."

Your TG:HDL ratio (as it is known) is calculated on a fasting lipid profile, and if not separated by your doctor is easy to calculate if you know your triglyceride value and your HDL value (both in the same measurement mg/dL or mmol).

Simply take the Triglyceride and divide by the HDL; the closer to 1 the better.

For example: If triglycerides = 120 mg/dL and HDL = 40 mg/dL, then 120 / 40 = 3.0.

A score of 3 is high and indicates an elevated risk of heart attack and stroke.

A score of 1 is great. Below one is fabulous.

A word of caution, whilst this is a generally good measurement, like many of the metrics here it does NOT necessarily mean that you won't have a heart attack.

For example, my TG:HDL ratio was 0.9 at the time I had a heart attack.

My triglycerides were low, but because I had another genetic issue, my risk in another area was so high that even with this ratio being so good my risk was high.

When analysed in conjunction with some of the other measurements for risk though it can rule out a problem.

This should be available in your GP blood test panel.

LP(a)

Nan's Chapter Summary: There is a molecule called LP(a), often referred to as LP "little" A. This molecule is a very sticky particle, that creates thick scar tissue inside artery walls when it tries to repair them, and creates blood clots that can block the arteries.

If you have genetically high LP(a) then you are at a significantly higher risk for heart disease.

Humans increased our development of LP(a) about the same time we lost the ability to produce our own vitamin C. Some scientists believe that LP(a) was increased by our bodies to create a "sticking plaster" for artery wall damage, to compensate for our inability to produce vitamin C, which protects our artery walls."

I have added a link to a CVD blood test panel that includes LP(a), from Smart Nutrition here,[17] as it is not available as a test from GP's currently.

This is the genetic factor that affects me, and many other people that are told heart attacks just "run in the family".

Dr Matthius Rath studied this particle extensively and describes it as;

"One of the most effective repair molecules in the artery wall" …that sounds good until he follows with… **"with ongoing vitamin deficiency it becomes one of the most dangerous risk factors for atherosclerosis."** (such as chronically low vitamin C, creating arterial wall damage)

The Framingham Heart Study, the largest CVD risk-factor study ever undertaken, showed that LP(a) is a **tenfold greater risk factor predictor than LDL or cholesterol.**

LP(a) is an LDL particle with an additional lipoprotein attached which makes it particularly "sticky" and which also resists he enzyme breaking down scar tissue.

Malcolm Kendrick describes the role of LP(a) very clearly in his book **A Statin Nation.**

"When cracks develop in blood vessels, LP(a) is attracted to them. LP(a) then links to proteins in the artery

---

[17] https://smartnutrition.co.uk/health-tests/comprehensive-cardiovascular-risk-assessment/cv-health-profile/

walls and binds them very tightly, forming a strong plug that holds back the bleeding."

"LP(a) not only plugs the gap, it also stops the blood clot that has been formed from being broken down."

This is where the problem lies. Although it is helping to strongly repair damage, LP(a) leaves a build-up of scar tissue which ultimately decreases the aperture of the artery. Narrowing artery walls and promoting clotting are clearly not good for blood flow.

LP(a) quantity is independent of HDL and LDL quantity....so even if both of these standard cholesterol measurements look OK in a blood test (as in my case) that doesn't get you off the hook as far as LP(a) is concerned!

You should test for LP(a) specifically.

Kendrick continues;

"LP(a) levels associate robustly and specifically with increased CVD risk. The association is continuous in shape without a threshold and does not depend on high levels of LDL or non-HDL cholesterol, or on the levels or presence of other cardiovascular risk factors."

In other words....high LP(a) is as strong a predictor that you will suffer a heart attack as you can get, and a simple blood test should show this.

GP's in the UK don't even test for LP(a).

In fact my GP didn't even know what it was!

Most GP's wouldn't know the relationship between LP(a), lysine, proline and vitamin C, or have read any of the data that you can access through Rath's book.

I have added a link to a CVD blood test panel that includes LP(a), from Smart Nutrition here.[18]

If you find that your LP(a) is high, then there is not much you can do to lower it significantly, but you can reduce it a little.

There are, however, a few things that you can do to help reduce LP(a) particle quantity a little, and also reduce its adhesion to your artery walls, both of which will reduce your overall risk.

To achieve this Matthius Rath and Linus Pauling recommend a daily intake of:

- 6,000 - 18,000 mg of vitamin C (up to 200 times the RDA, spread throughout the day, to the bowel tolerance of each individual)

- 2,000 mg Proline

- 2,000 - 6,000 mg Lysine

Daily supplementation with Niacin (500mg rising to 2g in dose) is also found to have a positive effect at reducing LP(a) levels by up to 30% to 40% in some individuals, according to a 2015 study.[19]

Additionally, a 2016 medical review[20] concluded that;

"CoQ10 supplementation was paralleled by a slight but significant reduction of plasma Lp(a), particularly in patients with Lp(a)≥ 30 mg/dL."

---

18 https://smartnutrition.co.uk/health-tests/comprehensive-cardiovascular-risk-assessment/cv-health-profile/

19 https://pubmed.ncbi.nlm.nih.gov/25936305/

20 https://pubmed.ncbi.nlm.nih.gov/26836888/

A 2010 study[21] called *Lipoprotein(a) as a cardiovascular risk factor: current status* concluded;

"We recommend screening for elevated Lp(a) in those at intermediate or high CVD/CHD risk, a desirable level <50 mg/dL as a function of global cardiovascular risk, and use of niacin for Lp(a) and CVD/CHD risk reduction."

LP-PLA2

Nan's Chapter Summary: LP-PLA2 is present in blood tests when arteries start to clog. This is a very strong predictor that you have started to develop heart disease. It is measured in the test for LP(a) above.

Lipoprotein-associated phospholipase (LP-PLA2) is an enzyme produced in the early stages of atherosclerotic plaque formation.

It promotes inflammation and plaque instability, and is a specific marker for vascular inflammation.

It reflects atherosclerosis disease activity rather than plaque burden, which is a significant indicator, given that the majority of heart attacks and sudden coronary deaths are attributable to plaque rupture at sites of only moderate stenosis.

In other words, this is a significant predictor of impending heart disease, in fact has been shown as a stronger predictor of heart attacks than HS-CRP, cholesterol, or any other independent markers.

It is even a strong predictor when other risk factors are absent.

---

[21]   https://pubmed.ncbi.nlm.nih.gov/20965889/

If this marker was measured more frequently, surprise heart attacks (remember that's 50% of all heart attacks) would not be much of a surprise at all.

LP-PLA2 levels are also included in many private comprehensive CVD blood tests, including the blood test highlighted above for LP(a).

Fasting Insulin

Nan's Chapter Summary: *High insulin is a sign of poor hormone balance, and can be a very significant factor in heart disease.*

High fasting insulin levels are a good indicator of insulin resistance, whether or not a patient shows glucose intolerance.

It is not a standard blood test that you receive from your GP, but you should ask for one.

You can buy test kits from companies like Hormone Lab UK.[22]

As you will have gathered by the amount of coverage in this book, insulin levels are extremely significant and will highlight a problem if they are elevated.

When Ivor Cummins, the host of *The Fat Emperor* podcast was asked "What predicts a 2nd heart attack in someone who has already had one?" He had a few clear facts to share.

"Total cholesterol and LDL had zero predictive power over 7 years. Hypertension had a 2 times factor of risk increase. High insulin had a 7 times factor of risk increase."

---

[22] https://hormonelab.co.uk/products/insulin-in-testing-kit-blood-spot

HbA1c

Nan's Chapter Summary: HbA1c is a blood test that will show your doctor what your average blood sugar levels have been like over the previous few months.

This could highlight a lifestyle issue and how your body is coping with excess sugar or carbohydrate in your diet.

HbA1c is a measure of your average blood glucose over the previous few months.

For people without diabetes, the normal range for the HbA1c is between 19 and 48 mmol/mol. Anything between 42 and 48 is considered borderline high and you are at increased risk for developing type 2 diabetes, and of course you are at increased risk of heart disease.

Because this test shows a trailing average in your blood, and because the red blood cells in your circulation last for around 3-4 months, dietary interventions may take some time to show up in reduction of these specific markers even though they may be having an immediate effect.

Any increases or decreases in your HbA1c will happen over a period of at least 6 weeks, so be patient but keep them moving lower over time by following the dietary and lifestyle interventions in the C.R.A.S.H. protocol.

ApoB

Nan's Chapter Summary: ApoB is a little transporter protein in your blood which helps your doctor to establish your heart disease risk when it is measured and compared with other markers, but independently it may not be something that is tested for initially.

ApoB (Apolipoprotein B) is the primary lipoprotein transporter of VLDL, Lp(a) and LDL particles.

In some people it is useful to measure ApoB and in others it seems to be a bit of a red-herring as a marker for heart disease risk.

For example, if you are insulin resistant, and have high inflammation, then elevated ApoB can be problematic, but if you are insulin sensitive and metabolically healthy with low inflammation, then you might find that a high-fat ketogenic diet actually slightly increases your ApoB, but it is not a problem.

It doesn't come as part of the standard, or even many specialist private blood tests in the UK currently, so you would probably only start to look at it if you were getting very deep into your blood markers, but hadn't found the root cause of any risk yet.

It does start to have some significance as an indicator of risk when calculated as a ratio with ApoA1 though (see below).

ApoA1

Nan's Chapter Summary: *ApoA1 is a little transporter protein in your blood which helps your doctor to establish your heart disease risk when it is measured and compared with other markers, but independently it may not be something that is tested for initially.*

As a major component of HDL transport, ApoA1 helps to clear fats, including cholesterol, from white blood cells.

Although, like ApoB, ApoA1 is not of much significance on its own, a 2011 study [23] concluded that in obese subjects (those with metabolic issues relating to insulin resistance);

"An ApoB/ApoA1 ratio increase indicated an increased risk of Coronary Heart Disease".

If you already have the markers that indicate insulin resistance and your ApoB/ApoA1 ratio is high, then you should look to make lifestyle interventions immediately to reduce your risk.

The ApoB/ApoA-1 Ratio is a Strong Predictor of Cardiovascular Risk[24] is a paper that explains how this ratio is a little more reliable than the somewhat similar LDL/HDL ratio for risk prediction.

Homocysteine, 25-Hydroxy Vitamin D, Vitamin B12

Nan's Chapter Summary: Homocysteine is part of the CVD test kit from Smart Nutrition, and may indicate risk of stroke and predict severity of stroke.

Dr Mark Hyman MD is the MD, director and founder of the Center for Functional Medicine and author of the book, *Eat Fat, Get Thin: Why the Fat We Eat Is the Key to Sustained Weight Loss and Vibrant Health*

He thinks this particular test is useful as it measures the levels of key heart-protective nutrients;

---

23   https://www.ncbi.nlm.nih.gov/pmc/articles/PMC3597070/

24   https://www.intechopen.com/books/lipoproteins-role-in-health-and-diseases/the-apob-apoa-t-ratio-is-a-strong-predictor-of-cardiovascular-risk

"Your homocysteine measures your folate status and should be between 6 and 8 micromoles per litre."

A clinical study in 2017[25] explored the relationship between acute ischaemic stroke (IS) and serum levels of homocysteine, vitamin B12, and D concluded that;

"Serum homocysteine, vitamin B12, and vitamin D levels are associated with baseline first-ever stroke severity."

"There is some evidence that early detection and management of these laboratory parameters may contribute both to primary and to secondary stroke prevention."

This is definitely a test that may prove useful. Homocysteine is part of the Smart Nutrition CVD blood test kit.

Ferritin

Nan's Chapter Summary: Iron is important in the body, but too much or too little can be problematic.

If your ferritin levels are rising they indicate that your iron levels are rising too, and this can significantly increase heart disease risk.

Too much iron can lead to life-threatening conditions, such as liver disease, heart problems and diabetes.

Iron is stored in a protein called ferritin in the body.

Iron is an important component of haemoglobin, the substance in red blood cells that carries oxygen from your lungs to transport it throughout your body.

---

[25]   https://www.ncbi.nlm.nih.gov/pmc/articles/PMC5382296/

Iron is essential for good heart health and low iron is a significant risk factor for heart disease, and can cause an irregular heartbeat.

Unfortunately, high iron levels are also problematic.

Optimum iron levels may boost heart health, but iron levels that are too high can increase risk of stroke.

Some studies suggested that the prevalence of atherosclerosis and insulin resistance is significantly increased with increasing ferritin levels.

A 2019 study [26] looked at the influence of serum ferritin on cardio-vascular risk factors, and found that;

"In conclusion, elevated ferritin level increased the risk of cardiovascular risk factors in first-degree relatives with family history of diabetes."

Most people don't need iron supplements unless recommended by a doctor, and iron levels are cumulative and excess iron is stored in our organs, especially our liver, heart and pancreas.

We can't secrete iron, so once we have too much iron in the body it would generally need to be either chelated-out or we would need a phlebotomy to remove it (in other words our blood is removed and replaced by blood with a lower concentration of iron).

Chelators are able to bind metal ions for drastic reduction in their reactivity, which can enter bloodstream and be excreted without any damage.

---

[26]
https://bmccardiovascdisord.biomedcentral.com/articles/10.1186/s12872-019-1068-5

Our main dietary sources of iron are generally noted as leafy green vegetables such as spinach and kale, and red meat.

There are two types of iron. Heme iron (found in red meat) and non-heme iron (found in leafy green vegetation).

If you are low in iron, supplementing your diet with non-heme iron is somewhat inefficient, because a large proportion of the iron is not bio-available, in other words your body can't use it.

In a ScienceDirect article[27] on how to avoid iron deficiency, the explanation of the absorption rates of the two types of iron was discussed.

"Heme iron is found in meat, fish, and poultry. 15–35% of heme iron is absorbed."

"Only 2–20% of nonheme iron is absorbed by the body, and absorption of nonheme iron is affected by a number of factors."

In general, normal ferritin levels range from 12 to 300 ng/mL of blood for males and 12 to 150 ng/mL for females.

Unless you know your iron is low, it is not recommended to supplement with iron, but to rely on dietary modifications to ensure iron is adequate but not too high.

Fibrinogen

Nan's Chapter Summary: Fibrinogen demonstrates that there is some inflammation in the body, and it also acts to clot blood.

High levels can be a significant indicator of heart disease.

---

[27] https://www.sciencedirect.com/topics/agricultural-and-biological-sciences/iron-absorption

Fibrinogen is an inflammatory marker, and it is also a clotting agent to prevent bleeding.

It is described as a "positive" acute-phase protein, so it's levels in the blood rise in response to systemic inflammation, tissue injury, and certain other events.

It is also elevated in certain cancers.

Elevated levels of fibrinogen in inflammation have been suggested to be the cause of thrombosis, and vascular injury that accompanies these conditions.

If your fibrinogen is high, then it follows that you are probably experiencing the double risks of blood clots and inflammation, so this is a significant potential marker for heart disease.

In The Quebec Cardiovascular Study, researchers concluded that;

"High fibrinogen levels associated with high Lp(a) levels significantly increased the risk of coronary heart disease."

A normal value for fibrinogen is between 200 and 400 mg/dL.

A fibrinogen value of less than 50 mg/dL may mean you're in danger of bleeding after surgery.

A fibrinogen value of more than 700 mg/dL may mean you're in danger of forming clots that could harm your heart or brain.

HS-CRP

Nan's Chapter Summary: HS-CRP *is an indicator that you have some inflammation in your system, and if this is persistent then you will be increasing your risk for heart disease.*

HS-CRP levels are shown on a standard GP blood test and most private blood test kits.

High Sensitivity - C Reactive Protein, is a measurement of inflammation in the body and as heart disease is primarily a disease caused by chronic inflammation. Elevated HS-CRP is a reason to take action.

It can be elevated by a wide variety of conditions such as burns, trauma, infections, pneumonia, tuberculosis, lupus, vasculitis, rheumatoid arthritis, inflammatory bowel disease and certain cancers.

If your levels of HS-CRP are not high it doesn't mean there is no cause for concern, this doesn't rule-out heart disease, but a high level should always be a strong warning signal to seek out and eradicate inflammation.

In a study from 2000[28] conducted on 28,263 apparently healthy postmenopausal women (over a mean follow-up period of three years) to assess the risk of cardiovascular events, HS-CRP was proven significant;

"Of the 12 markers measured, HS-CRP was the strongest predictor of the risk of cardiovascular events."

Other risk factors measured included serum amyloid A, interleukin-6, and soluble intercellular adhesion molecule type 1 (sICAM-1), homocysteine and a variety of lipid and lipoprotein measurements.

---

[28]   https://pubmed.ncbi.nlm.nih.gov/10733371/

An HS-CRP level less than 1 mg/L will put you at low-risk for CVD from an inflammation standpoint alone.

An HS-CRP level between 1 mg/L and 3 mg/L will put you at medium-risk for CVD from an inflammation standpoint alone.

An HS-CRP level greater than 3 mg/L is a sign of infection, trauma or chronic disease, and will put you at high-risk for CVD from an inflammation standpoint alone.

As mentioned before though, low HS-CRP does not mean you have no risk, it just means you have low inflammation.

My HS-CRP was less than 1, but because I had very high LP(a) I was still at a significant heart disease risk, even with low inflammation.

HOMA-IR

Nan's Chapter Summary: HOMA-IR *is a test you can calculate yourself from the link below.*

This is a test to let you know if you are struggling to manage your hormone, insulin.

If the levels are high this can indicate that you may be on a path towards type 2 diabetes, and it may increase your heart disease risk.

HOMA-IR stands for Homeostatic Model Assessment of Insulin Resistance.

I have mentioned "insulin resistance" quite a bit because it is one of, if not the most important feature of modern chronic disease.

This measurement demonstrates the presence and extent of any insulin resistance.

HOMA-IR is calculated thus; fasting insulin (microU/L) x fasting glucose (mmol/L) divided by 22.5

There is a link to a HOMA-IR calculator here [29], but you will need your glucose (mg/dL) numbers and your insulin (mU/L) numbers from your blood test for the calculation.

As an indication, below 1 is great, 1-2 is OK, above 2 and you have a bit of a problem!

Insulin resistance is reversable through dietary and lifestyle interventions, and you can make quite a big difference to your insulin sensitivity quite quickly when adopting some of the strategies outlined in this book.

Leptin

Nan's Chapter Summary: Leptin is a hormone that makes us feel full-up after eating.

This hormone can work with other hormones to promote issues with our metabolism, and cause inflammation.

This would not be on a standard test, but if a person that had suffered with heart disease couldn't find the cause elsewhere, they may want to check leptin levels.

Leptin is a funny little hormone.

Leptin plays a pivotal role in the regulation of energy stability, neuroendocrine function, and metabolism in not only states of energy excess but, more importantly, in states of energy deficiency.

It is known primarily for making us feel satiated...or "full-up".

---

[29]   https://www.thebloodcode.com/homa-ir-calculator/

In other words, it has the opposite effect of the hormone ghrelin, which makes us feel hungry.

A review of research on Leptin entitled *The Role of Leptin in Human Physiology* [30] from 2010 stated that;

"Leptin deficiency is a clinical syndrome associated with distinct phenotypes, which encompass a very small subset of obesity."

There is some interesting research in a study entitled *Leptin and Cardiovascular Disease* [31] published in 2008, on the different ways that leptin levels can influence inflammation and heart disease, and the mechanisms where one might become leptin resistant (in much the same way as we can become insulin resistant).

"The ability of leptin to promote proinflammatory signaling through cytokines and growth factors may contribute to endothelial dysfunction, atherosclerosis, and insulin resistance in hyperleptinemic states."

Higher leptin equals higher inflammatory state so higher risk for vascular inflammation.

This is unlikely to be a test that you will receive from a doctor, and would not be one to request unless you have exhausted all other avenues and not found your root-cause for disease.

Particle Size

---

[30]   https://www.ncbi.nlm.nih.gov/pmc/articles/PMC2829242/

[31]

   https://www.ahajournals.org/doi/full/10.1161/circulationaha.107.741645

Nan's Chapter Summary: In the section What Causes Heart Disease, I mentioned that particle size of cholesterol molecules is a potential risk-factor, and there are some tests that you can take to establish your particle size.

This doesn't yet form part of a standard GP test, but I think it should.

The Smart Nutrition blood test mentioned earlier provides details of cholesterol particle size.

Whilst HDL and LDL are not measurements I would particularly worry about from a CVD risk perspective, I would recommend getting your particle size checked.

As mentioned earlier in the book, particle size is a risk factor for atherosclerosis risk, and is genetically determined for each of us.

Having said this, lifestyle, particularly diet can influence particle size.

It is worth repeating, that the most important actions you can take to positively impact your LDL and HDL profile, is not to reduce them or remove them….***it is to optimise them, increase the ratio of HDL to LDL and improve the particle sizes of both of them.***

This is achieved by eating more saturated fat, and less sugar!

A letter [32] in the British Medical Journal in 2013, by retired GP Madhvi Chanrai, referred to the work of Dr Malhotra on the subject of cholesterol particle size, and thanked him for his contribution to the subject and his brave publication of the unpopular truth when it stated;

---

[32]   https://www.bmj.com/content/347/bmj.f6340/rr/669222

"It was thoroughly gratifying to read the following key points in Dr Malhotra's article:

1) Dietary carbohydrates increase levels of highly atherogenic small, dense LDL cholesterol.

2) Dietary saturated fat increases levels of both HDL cholesterol (which is inversely correlated with cardiovascular disease) and large buoyant LDL cholesterol (which is known not to be atherogenic)."

He continued:

"For many years we have been unwittingly giving incorrect advice to our patients – from the 70's onwards we told them to cut down on eggs and other cholesterol rich foods (it has now been known for many years that dietary cholesterol does in fact reduce levels of small LDL particles); and that they should eat margarine instead of butter (at that time unbeknownst to us margarine used to be full of trans fats, and now they are full of pro-inflammatory omega-6 PUFAs)."

"It will take many years to convince the general public that dietary cholesterol and saturated fat are not the villains that they were once purported to be, and that it is in fact sugar, bread, rice, pasta, and sweet drinks (including juices and smoothies) that we should be avoiding instead of fat. We need to urgently start undoing the harm that we have done with the dietary advice that has been meted out over the last few decades."

His summary is worthy of a diagram, so I have included it here:

UNCONVENTIONAL
WISDOM

- FOOD IS NOT JUST A SIMPLE FUEL – IT IS ALSO A TYPE OF ENVIRONMENTAL EXPOSURE.
- PROPER NUTRITION OFFERS ONE OF THE CHEAPEST AND MOST EFFECTIVE WAYS OF DECREASING THE RISK OF CARDIOVASCULAR DISEASE AND MANY OTHER WESTERN DISEASES, INCLUDING OBESITY.
- SMALL, DENSE LDL PARTICLES ARE PARTICULARLY ATHEROGENIC.
- SMALL, DENSE LDL PARTICLES ARE CORRELATED WITH CARBOHYDRATE INTAKE.
- FRUCTOSE INCREASES LEVELS OF SMALL, DENSE LDL MORE THAN GLUCOSE.
- SATURATED FAT INCREASES LEVELS OF HDL CHOLESTEROL.
- SATURATED FAT INCREASES LEVELS OF LARGE BUOYANT LDL CHOLESTEROL.
- A CALORIE TO ME ISN'T THE SAME AS A CALORIE TO YOU, BECAUSE WE BOTH METABOLISE THEM DIFFERENTLY.
- CHRONIC LOW-GRADE INFLAMMATION IS A KEY STEP IN MOST WESTERN DISEASES.
- THE RATIO OF OMEGA 6 TO OMEGA 3 IS CRUCIAL TO THE DEVELOPMENT OF INFLAMMATION.
- THE CURRENT OBESITY EPIDEMIC IN WESTERN COUNTRIES MIGHT NOT BE ONLY ABOUT 'TOO MUCH FOOD AND TOO LITTLE EXERCISE'; IT IS PROBABLY ALSO DUE TO A COMPLEX INTERACTION BETWEEN GENETICS, EPIGENETICS, AND THE MICROBIOTA
- CEREAL GRAINS PROMOTE AN INFLAMMATORY MICROBIOTA & LEPTIN RESISTANCE

NB: Transcript from a letter to the British Medical Journal in 2013 by then retired GP Madhvi Chapra:
https://www.bmj.com/content/347/bmj.f634/rr/662932

@ s e a n f a n e

Part 4: What Can You Do To Minimise Risk?

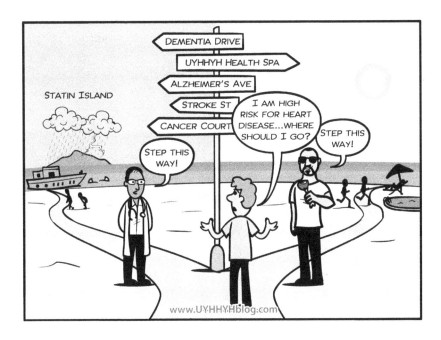

UNDERSTAND YOUR RESULTS

For most people it may require some investigation to really under-stand your risk profile for heart disease, but if you are a man over 40 and a woman over 50, even if you have no family history of heart disease and no reason to think you might be at risk, I would strongly recommend that you go through a series of tests to check your susceptibility.

If you do have a family history then I would recommend testing for genetic factors regardless of age, the sooner you know of a genetic issue, the sooner you can adapt your lifestyle to prevent it from becoming a problem.

Remember, 50% of heart attacks happen to people with no symp-toms or traditional risk-factors.

This doesn't mean that there aren't any risk-factors!

It just means that the traditional risk-factors that your doctor might evaluate (cholesterol, family history, obesity and smoking) may look OK, but there could be a significant risk-factor that they haven't tested for, such as the ones mentioned above.

A calcium CT scan for all men at 40 and all women at 50 should be a standard screening just as cervical smear tests and prostate tests are.

Until they become cheap enough to be a standard test, I would sug-gest you organise one as soon as you hit those ages, if it is affordable for you, or as soon as you can thereafter.

They are a 'nailed-on' view of current heart disease progression and prediction of a future heart attack.

If, after testing, you would like help understanding your risk factors then please contact your test company, and they should be able to direct you to the professional resources to understand your results.

Eradicate Risk Where You Can

Once we understand our risk profile we will have a list of areas where we can focus our attention, to mitigate any risk.

This will probably consist of a few lifestyle, hormonal and environmental factors and possibly some genetic factors that we will want to address.

The lifestyle and hormonal elements can often be remedied with simple interventions or supplements.

Many of these are highlighted in the next part of this book.

The genetic factors might take a little more care and attention.

UNDERSTAND GENETIC FACTORS THAT YOU CAN'T CONTROL

We can't control our genetics.

We can, however, do things that either prevent negative genetic traits from expressing themselves, or mitigate against the negative effects that are expressed, so we should never feel that we are blighted by a fate that we have no ability to positively influence.

It may be harder for some people than others, and that may seem unfair, but there is almost always something, or a number of things that we can do to positively impact our health….regardless of the poor hand our genetic croupier may have dealt us.

So don't get too downhearted about a genetic issue…….just be a little more persistent about how to deal with it.

FORMULATE A PLAN

Lastly, we will need to formulate a plan.

We can't get to the stage where we have heart disease and expect that we will instantly feel capable of understanding our risk, alter our lifestyle and mitigate any genetic challenge without a plan.

If you are worried about your heart health, then this book provides information to help you to formulate a plan that can help with adapting to changes that will hopefully transform your health, and mitigate your risk.

LIFESTYLE HABITS TO HEAL YOUR HEART - & HOW TO STICK TO THEM

THE C.R.A.S.H. PROGRAMME

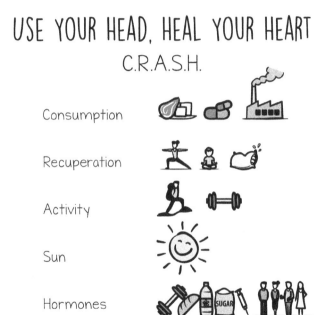

USE YOUR HEAD, HEAL YOUR HEART
C.R.A.S.H.

Consumption

Recuperation

Activity

Sun

Hormones

Nan's Chapter Summary: *This is my C.R.A.S.H. course in heart health.*

I created this acronym to make it easy to remember the 5 elements that can dramatically reduce heart disease risk and improve recovery for those that have already experienced heart disease.

Each letter in C.R.A.S.H. stands for a different part of the lifestyle, diet and supplementary areas that you can adjust, or adapt, to dramatically reduce your heart disease risk.

They may also help to reverse any CVD that you already have, if the diet and lifestyle changes are adopted whole-heartedly.

CONSUMPTION

Regardless of your underlying conditions, the lifestyle options outlined in my C.R.A.S.H. formula are designed to optimise your cardio-vascular health, and create robust protection from CVD.

The *C* in C.R.A.S.H. is Consumption.

I explained how oxidation, inflammation and hormone imbalances are fuelled by the various foods we eat, the particles we breathe, the substances we absorb physically and the thoughts we accept and nurture.

All of these areas of consumption can be negative, or positive, for our health.

Here are some ways that we can adapt our consumption to improve our heart health.

Diet

Nan's Chapter Summary: We consume things in a number of ways, as has been discussed in the chapters earlier about the causes of heart disease.

The first form of consumption is our diet. What we eat can either promote or prevent heart disease. If we eat heavily processed foods, seed oils and sugar and starch, we promote the hormone imbalances and inflammation in our body to promote heart disease.

If we eat a diet rich in high-quality sources of protein, good fats (such as avocado, coconut oil, fatty fish, eggs, cheese, milk and red meat) then we will create more hormonal balance and we will improve our immune system.

Additionally, vegetables and fruits with a low glycemic load will provide additional nutrients, but will not promote hormonal imbalance.

It is very important that the food that you eat is high quality. Whilst they are a little more expensive, grass-fed beef, organic free-range eggs, wild caught salmon and organic vegetables are all examples of products that have a dramatically improved nutrient content than cheaper alternatives.

Our diet is one of the most easily influenceable, and powerful interventions we can make to cure ourselves from chronic disease.

Everything we put in our mouths will either have a positive or negative impact on our physical and mental wellbeing.

This impact may not always be obvious at the time we eat or drink something, but if you think of your body as an engine, what you put into it will either help it to run perfectly, or result in a mechanical issue at some point.

If we put a teaspoon of water into the full petrol tank of our car, we may not notice any issue with it initially.

If we did this every day, then it would be likely that we would irreparably damage the engine within 2 months.

We would never dream of putting anything other than fuel in our cars, and we would think anybody that did, and who damaged their engine as a result, as pretty dumb I should think.

We put oil in the oil sump to lubricate the engine. We never add other substances instead, out of convenience.

If after having our car serviced, the mechanic told us that he had reused some old pond water for the cooling system because it was cheaper, added some vodka into the anti-freeze because the bottle was beside the car and poured vegetable oil into the sump for lubrication because it looked similar to motor oil, we would be mortified, but we take this approach to fuelling our bodies every day.

When it comes to our bodies, most of us just eat or drink whatever tastes nice, or is convenient, or is cheap.

The reality is, despite the fact that we may not see the effects of doing this straight away, like the spoonful of water in the petrol tank, the damage that is done to our bodies from constantly feeding ourselves poor quality fuel, or worse still toxic substances bearing no relation to food, will accumulate until our own unique ability to tolerate it any more is reached and then we will suffer the consequences.

Some of these consequences are easy to spot and are reversible.

Gaining weight is one of these consequences. We can see it happening bit-by-bit, we can survive gaining some weight for a while with limited negative impact, and in most cases we can reverse weight gain and repair most or all of the damage that being in an obese state had caused, as soon as we address the dietary issues.

The same is not true of many chronic diseases.

In many cases the damage is being caused steadily, over a long period of time, and until the consequences become very obvious there may be no gradually worsening symptoms.

Heart disease is very much like this.

In most cases, one would not notice the steady build-up of atherosclerosis.

Some people have no symptoms or prior warning before a heart attack.

Some have mild angina (pressing feeling in the upper abdomen or middle of the chest), which can be easily mistaken for indigestion or other gastric complaint.

When symptoms do appear, it is generally when an artery is already over 70% blocked[1], which would means atherosclerosis would be quite advanced.

So, with modern chronic diseases, if we are lucky, we are able to reverse any damage we have created, but in some cases the damage may be irreversible and the outcome may be a lifetime of poor health and medication or worse, an early death.

This is the future awaiting many of us, according to the statistics.

Most of us will die from a preventable chronic disease.

"Each year roughly 10 million people die from cancer, and nearly 20 million die from heart disease around the world. Another 50 million have Alzheimer's, and almost half a billion of us have diabetes." says Ben Bikman in Why We Get Sick.

Our diet should provide us with, not just energy, but the macronutrients to thrive and the vitamins and micronutrients to optimise our body's potential, to enable our organs to function, our immune system to protect us and our cells to repair and grow.

This may seem obvious, but it is really easy to be confused by dietary regimes, and many don't provide great nutrient density or variety.

There are so many different eating styles and patterns that can be undertaken, and there are many commercial organisations or individuals that will promote one over another to gain a commercial benefit.

---

[1]   https://myheart.net/articles/heart-blockage-explained-with-pictures/

I want you to understand the principles of how to eat, so you can make better choices for yourself, and use this information to improve your heart health and repair your cardiovascular system.

I would not advocate a prescriptive diet plan where you weigh and measure all your food and track your "macros" in an app, and I absolutely don't want to advocate you becoming food obsessed.

There are, however, a few key principles and concepts to understand.

Managing Insulin is one of these.

Managing your body's production of insulin is one of the cornerstones of good dietary health, and it is easy to do when you are experienced at it, but it can be challenging to make the adjustment to it initially.

The best way this is achieved, is by choosing to eat foods with a lower glycemic load.

If you eat to minimise your circulating blood glucose, which in-turn reduces insulin, this is referred to as a ketogenic diet.

It is called ketogenic, because rather than using glucose as an energy source, the body uses molecules called ketones which are produced by the liver.

Ketone production is increased when there is limited glucose and, therefore, low insulin.

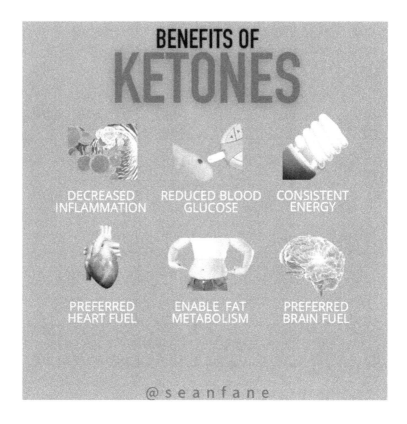

If we have periods of time when we don't eat at all (for example when we skip breakfast and have our first meal of the day at lunchtime) the extended period of time with no food will lower our blood glucose, and we will start to create more ketones for energy.

We all have ketones to a lesser or greater degree all the time.

Being on a ketogenic diet is particularly useful for a number of reasons, some of which make weight loss easier.

As anyone who has tried to lose weight will know, appetite can become a significant factor in the weight loss process.

Twenty-five years ago, the only known appetite-controlling hormone was insulin.

When blood insulin levels are high, glucose is stored as glycogen and deposited into fat cells. This results in a reduction of circulating fuel, which stimulates appetite.

You may recognise the experience of being hungry 2-3 hours after eating a high carbohydrate, low fat meal.

Many people contend that increased insulin is the dominant signal that makes us become obese, but in the interim we have discovered many other circulating, cellular signals that communicate the body's energy status and regulate appetite and metabolism.

Among these regulatory hormones are leptin and ghrelin.

Both have receptors in the brain that transmit their biochemical message into behaviour – leptin tells us to "eat less" and ghrelin tells us to "eat more".

When you adhere to a ketogenic diet this changes dramatically for the better.

Blood insulin levels go down. The satiety hormone leptin also goes down, but the brain's sensitivity to leptin increases dramatically when on a ketogenic diet.

Lasting weight loss results can be achieved, without purposeful calorie restriction, or the need to resist persistent hunger, and are associated with long-term adherence to a ketogenic diet [2].

In other words, with a ketogenic diet the brain perceives a greater satiety response to less leptin, so we feel less hungry.

---

[2]   https://www.virtahealth.com/blog/ketosis-appetite-hunger

Another key factor, in ketogenic diets favour, comes from the fact that that the brain's response to leptin is inhibited by inflammation[3].

This results in leptin resistance.

We know that inflammation is dramatically reduced by sustained nutritional ketosis [4], so it appears that the reduction in leptin resistance, due to reduced inflammation, more than compensates for the lower leptin levels [5].

This reduction in inflammation and increase in sensitivity to leptin, together with the reduced blood insulin levels characteristic of ketosis, can explain why we see a decrease in appetite on a sustained ketogenic diet.

As Ben Bikman describes in *Why We Get Sick*;

"Not only are ketones recognised as a valuable fuel source for almost every cell, including the brain and muscles, but they're also important signalling molecules."

"Some of the known benefits of ketones include reducing oxidative stress and controlling inflammation."

Clearly these are two very powerful reasons why ketogenic diets are extremely important for a person that has experienced heart disease, as oxidation and inflammation are the catalysts for atherosclerosis.

An additional benefit in adapting to using mainly ketones for energy, is that our bodies can utilise stored fat as energy very efficiently

---

[3]   https://pubmed.ncbi.nlm.nih.gov/25589226/

[4]   https://pubmed.ncbi.nlm.nih.gov/18046594/

[5]   https://pubmed.ncbi.nlm.nih.gov/29712560/

when we are in a ketogenic "state", and the absence of insulin means fat cells can release their energy stores.

This inevitably means weight-loss is accelerated through utilising body-fat for energy.

This doesn't happen when we eat a diet rich in carbohydrates, because these foods stimulate the production of insulin, which then "locks" the fat cells, preventing them from being utilised as energy.

A further unique advantage of a ketogenic diet for weight-loss is how our bodies deal with excess energy capacity.

When we eat a normal diet that increases blood glucose, any excess glucose is shuttled into fat cells by insulin, and when we have a deficit if glucose, hormones signal us to eat more, so we can become quite hungry, creating the potential to over-eat and therefore create more fat storage.

When we eat a ketogenic diet, any excess ketones can be **wasted** by the body which expels them in the urine and in our breath, and when we have a deficit our liver can either make more, or, because there is no insulin keeping fat cells locked, we can open fat cells in our body and use our body's own energy stores.

This is essentially how humans have evolved to produce energy for hundreds of thousands of years, before the agricultural revolution and the development of processed food meant that we had a diet of nearly 80% carbohydrates and sugar.

Finally, ketones are the preferred fuel source for the brain, and ketogenic diets are now being used to great effect in treating a variety of cognitive (brain) issues, such as Alzheimer's, dementia, memory loss, cognitive impairment, epilepsy and autism.

A review in 2014 [6] stated that;

"The ketogenic diet is a therapy for multiple forms of epilepsy in both children and adults. The utility of this diet for the treatment of a variety of neurodegenerative disorders suggests common central mechanisms that restore imbalances in energy metabolism."

Insulin resistance of the brain associated with Alzheimer's is so well documented that Alzheimer's is often referred to as *"type 3 diabetes"*. [7]

This brain insulin resistance may help explain why those with type 2 diabetes have higher rates of Alzheimer's [8].

A 2004 study [9] revealed that 81% of people with Alzheimer's had either type 2 diabetes or pre-diabetes.

In another study [10], people who died with Alzheimer's disease had evidence of brain glucose dysregulation.

---

[6]   https://www.jlr.org/article/S0022-2275(20)34975-0/fulltext

[7]   https://pubmed.ncbi.nlm.nih.gov/25088942/

[8]   https://pubmed.ncbi.nlm.nih.gov/29950970/

[9]   https://pubmed.ncbi.nlm.nih.gov/14747300/

[10] https://pubmed.ncbi.nlm.nih.gov/29055815/

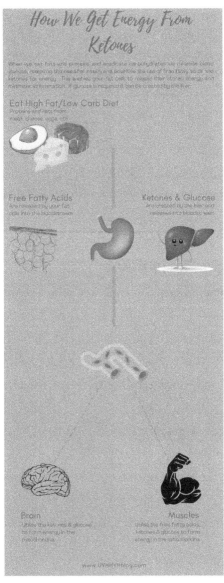

So providing ketones to your brain for fuel, instead of glucose seems to be preferable for optimal cognitive function, and to reduce the likelihood and the impact of a number of cognitive impairments.

When we eat a diet high in fats (particularly good saturated and monounsaturated fats) and protein, but very low in carbohydrates, we can gain the maximum benefit from ketone molecules, reduce inflammation, manage insulin, create stable and consistent energy, experience reduced hunger and cravings and become much more mentally alert.

When you think about food, think about getting clean!

Eat foods that you recognise as a natural food product.

Try to ensure that your food has been grown (or raised) with the minimum levels of human intervention from "advanced" agricultural practices.

Local, free-range, grass-fed, humanely treated, beef.

Wild-caught, Alaskan salmon.

Local fruit and vegetables with minimum use of pesticides and machinery.

All of these choices make a massive cumulative difference to your health.

Learn to cook so you can choose the ingredients that support your health.

Avoid sugar, vegetable oils, processed foods, snacks (protein bars, crisps, nachos, sweets).

These are the antithesis of food, and in many cases are actually low-dose poison.

Minimise high GL (glycemic-load), genetically modified grains and starches such as potatoes, wheat, corn and rice. These damage your hormone balance, and hormones rule everything!

If you are already low-risk and want to prevent becoming high-risk for heart disease, then I would say minimising high GL foods and being very active will be pretty much the bulk of your job done.

If you are already high-risk, then I would strongly advise something akin to a ketogenic diet, where you essentially remove foods that elevate insulin from your shopping list entirely.

Want to stay well?

Get Clean! (with your food)

Intermittent Fasting

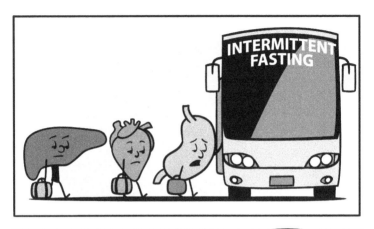

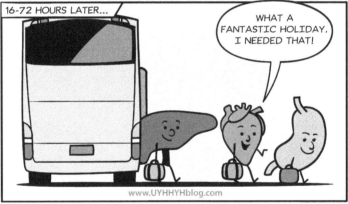

Nan's Chapter Summary: *When we go for periods without eating, our bodies start a repair process, and the hormones responsible for managing our digestion and metabolism recover and rest.*

Short periods of fasting, like for 18 hours (or a day) can significantly improve the management of blood sugar and reduce heart disease risk and blood pressure.

It's not just what we eat, but when we eat that can have a big impact on our health.

Not much more than 30 years ago, most adults and children had daily meals separated by 5 hours, today this has been reduced to three and half (on average), and that is without snacking between meals (something that was less frequent back then).

Adults also consume, on average, 400 calories more per day[11] (once snacks are factored in) than in the early 1980's (United States data).

Eating carbohydrate-rich diets full of wheat, grains, starches and sugars will elevate glucose and insulin for a good few hours after each meal, right up to our next meal or snack. It is easy to see how every waking moment our bodies could be exposed to elevated blood glucose and elevated insulin.

Friedrich Nietzsche said in 1888 *"What doesn't kill you makes you stronger."* and he was right if what he meant was that some form of adversity or stress is important to stimulate growth and repair.

Here is a great example. In order to build muscle, we must first damage muscle fibres. We do this voluntarily with resistance training.....lifting weights literally tears our muscle fibres.

Our body responds by repairing the damaged fibres, and in the process creates stronger muscles. This is an example of a type of stress referred to as hormesis.

Hormesis describes the beneficial effect of low-level stressors.

---

[11]   https://academic.oup.com/ajcn/article/91/5/1342/4597335

Hormesis is good stress, as opposed to chronic, long-term stress from things like a demanding job, financial worries, unstable relationships, grief, and other factors which can wreck our health.

Short-term or mild stressors can have a very positive effect.

Another example of a hormetic stressor is limiting the time in which we eat each day, which leaves longer gaps between consuming food. This is often referred to as intermittent fasting.

There are some fascinating studies looking at fasting and how it causes our bodies to activate protective mechanisms for our short-term survival, which benefit our health and lifespan.

If we are constantly in a state of calorie abundance, our bodies become lazy. When we remove food security, our biology wakes-up and starts to act.

"Fasting" is any time we are not eating....hence break*fast*, being the break of the fast we have had whilst we have been asleep.

One of the reasons our bodies can do so much good work repairing and replenishing whilst we sleep, is that we aren't using lots of resources for digesting and processing what we put in our mouths.

A "fast" that lasts longer than our 8-ish hour sleep has many additional benefits, such as:

- Reducing blood glucose

- Increasing growth hormone (HGH) - which helps boost muscle growth, strength and helps us recover from injury and disease

- Reducing inflammation - fasting reduces monocytes in the blood, and reduces oxidative stress in cells

- Reducing body fat - your body adapts to using fat cells and ketones for energy, instead of carbohydrates from food after about 16 hours

- Autophagy - an extremely beneficial, internal, cellular "spring-cleaning" process where your body recycles damaged cells

A "fast" can be as long as one feels comfortable with, but the benefits increase with the duration of the fast, until they seem to peak at 72 hours without food, after which they start to decline.

Intermittent fasting, eating within a restricted time window, is a great way to get some of the benefits above.

A common practice for those that enjoy intermittent fasting is to eat between Noon and 8pm. This means going from 8pm to the following day at noon (16 hours) without food.

This enables access to most of the health benefits of fasting to some degree.

Personally, I don't really eat until about 2pm, and probably have my last meal between 8pm and 9pm.

Periodically adding a 24, 48 or 72 hour fast (maybe every month or two) really accelerates these benefits.

Additionally, people who fast for 24 hours at least once a month are shown to be half as likely to be insulin resistant [12] as those that don't.

---

[12]   https://pubmed.ncbi.nlm.nih.gov/22425331/

"A reported fasting association with a lower CAD risk was also validated and fasting associations with lower glucose and BMI were found".

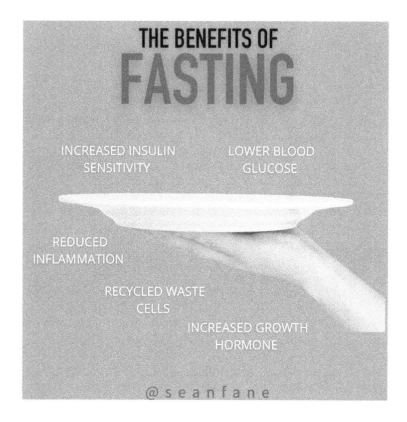

I have experimented with many different types of eating "window" and fasting patterns, but I find the following system works really well for me:

The first Monday of each month I start a 3 day fast....so I will eat dinner on the first Wednesday night of each month, with my previous meal having been dinner on the previous Sunday.

Every remaining Monday of the month I will eat one meal that day at 8pm-ish.

On all other days I eat my first meal of the day at about 2pm and my last by 9pm.

Think you might get too hungry doing the same? Surprisingly you probably won't (well not if you are already on a ketogenic diet or have got used to eating in a restricted window......it can be difficult when you first try it though).

When I first started fasting I noticed that after a relatively challenging first 24 hours, as my body adapted to the change in incoming fuel source, I actually started to feel great, and lose feelings of hunger, as ghrelin levels (the hormone responsible for making you hungry) decreased.

When I was younger, I ate a lot, and I ate from the moment I woke up to the moment I went to bed.

I was constantly hungry (hangry even) and would feel either hyperactive after a meal or crash through the floor with very low energy soon afterwards.

I was extremely active playing sport, and was very slim, and fit, but unhealthy.

What I now know, is that I was suffering from the challenges one faces with a continual flow of glucose, creating constantly elevated insulin, and the subsequent hyperglycaemic and hypoglycaemic challenges that this brings.

I couldn't go three hours without food, or I felt awful.

Having experimented for a few years now with intermittent fasting, I am amazed at how I barely even remember to eat some days, and have a very steady balance of energy. It is very common for my partner Julie to need to remind me to eat something.

I feel completely alert, energetic and happy without ever really giving food a second thought throughout a normal day.

It's not like I am inactive either…I start the day with yoga and some callisthenics or weights, then walk the dogs and most days also go for a 2 hour lunchtime walk with Julie covering roughly 17,000 steps, before returning for breakfast at 2pm.

I literally could not imagine even sitting at a desk and reaching 10am without food a few years ago. It would have seemed impossible.

One of the biggest benefits of fasting is increased autophagy. Autophagy literally means "self-eating," but don't worry, this is a good thing, as you will discover.

Our cells are continually being damaged through natural processes, such as performing immune functions, energy conversion and digestion.

With age, stress, exposure to food and chemicals, our cells experience something called free-radical damage. This damages them at a faster rate than usual, and as a result our bodies need a process to remove these damaged cells.

There is, however, a cellular "life-cycle", where new cells are generated to help the body perform optimally, and old cells are removed at the same time. This is autophagy.

Without autophagy, remaining damaged cells can trigger inflammation in the body and lead to the development of diseases.

Whilst autophagy is a function that happens to a small degree throughout the day, this activity significantly increases after 16 hours without food.

You don't need to feel like you are starving yourself in order to generate the benefits of autophagy, but leaving at least 12-16 hours as a daily fast certainly helps to keep this process working well. This is easily done by just "skipping" breakfast.

Autophagy plays a role in our longevity too.

We humans have evolved to live longer thanks to our ability to respond to biological stressors, like physical activity and famine, and our ancestors immune systems adapted over time in order to survive.

A study from Newcastle University[13] discovered that this ability is due to small adaptations in a protein known as p62, which is the key to starting the autophagy process in the body.

The activation of p62 takes place when your body senses the presence of reactive oxygen species, the metabolic by-products that cause cell damage.

P62 proteins work to remove damage that has accumulated in your body so that you're better equipped to handle biological stress. Homeostasis and vibrant health are a direct result of p62 protein activity during autophagy.

The autophagic process of removing damaged cells' interior organelles and replacing them with new ones is what keeps you healthy.

"Sensing stress and activating protective processes like autophagy, may have evolved to allow better stress resistance and a longer lifespan." says the study's lead author Dr. Viktor Korolchuk.

If, periodically, you feel like fasting, then these benefits will be available to you:

- Reduced inflammation
- Disease prevention

---

13   https://www.sciencedaily.com/releases/2018/01/180118114139.htm

- Increased longevity

- Protection of the nervous system

- Protection of the immune system

- Protection against metabolic stress

- Encouragement of new cell growth (especially those in the brain and heart tissue, enhancing cognitive function and protecting against heart disease)

- Improved digestive function (by repairing the gut lining)

- Protection of genes (by maintaining the integrity and stability of DNA)

- Suppression of tumours in some cancers

Here are some tips on how to kick-start autophagy:

1. **Eat a High-Fat/Low-Carb (ketogenic) diet** - This makes transitioning to intermittent fasting much easier. According to Naomi Whittel, author of the autophagy-centric book *Glow15: A Science-Based Plan to Lose Weight, Revitalize Your Skin, and Invigorate Your Life "Fat needs to be the dominant macronutrient in our diets because it's different from protein. Whereas protein can become a sugar, fat cannot."*

2. **Intermittent Fasting** – Research[14] suggests that autophagy and fasting go hand in hand, as you can ramp up the autophagic

---

[14]   https://www.ncbi.nlm.nih.gov/pmc/articles/PMC3106288/

process by limiting your eating window, or skipping breakfast. Best results are achieved with a slightly longer fast though.

3. **Sleep** - A 2016 study[15] suggests that autophagy follows circadian rhythms, and that sleep interruptions seem to disrupt autophagy, so good sleep helps the process.

Another great benefit from fasting is an increase in secretion of HGH (Human Growth Hormone).

HGH fuels childhood growth, but also helps maintain tissues and organs throughout life.

HGH deficiency in adults leads to higher levels of body fat, lower lean body mass (sarcopenia) and decreased bone mass (osteopenia).

HGH is produced by the pituitary gland at the base of the brain, however, the pituitary gland slowly reduces the amount of growth hormone it produces as we age.

---

[15] https://www.tandfonline.com/doi/abs/10.3109/07420528.2015.11 37581

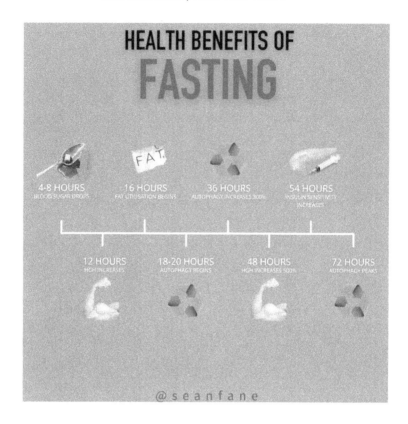

A 1988 study [16] explains how HGH secretion is amplified when fasting.

Low levels of HGH may facilitate loss of muscle and bone mass, so increasing this hormone as we age is extremely valuable.

16 https://www.ncbi.nlm.nih.gov/pmc/articles/PMC329619/

A study in 1990 in a New England Journal of Medicine article [17] tested the effects of giving HGH to older adults that had abnormally low levels.

Over a 6 month period, the group given HGH added 3.7 kg more lean mass, and their fat mass decreased an extra 2.4 kg when compared with the control group!

Additionally their skin thickness improved.

Results like this are why HGH is considered anti-ageing, as it seems to reverse some of the negative physical effects that we consider normal in our fifties and onwards.

Fasting is your friend if you are at high-risk for heart disease.

Gut Bacteria

Nan's Chapter Summary: *We have an abundance of good bacteria in our gut, and they help to boost our immune system, digest foods and fight against invaders or toxins.*

If these bacteria are not kept healthy, we are more susceptible to allergies, viruses and illness, as well as heart disease.

These bacteria are negatively affected by stress, high sugar foods and toxic substances. They are positively affected by high fibre foods and fermented foods.

They can also be damaged by antibiotics, so it is wise to avoid antibiotics wherever it is possible, and sensible, to do so.

---

[17]   https://pubmed.ncbi.nlm.nih.gov/2355952/

Unlike environmental bacteria, which we try to avoid for good health, our gut bacteria is incredibly important for our health, probably much more important than you think.

The gut microbiota, as they are sometimes called, are the trillions of microbes inhabiting the human intestine, a complex ecological community that through its collective metabolic activities, influence both physiology and disease susceptibility.

Our bodies are made up of both good and bad bacteria, and collectively, they form a delicate, and easily unbalanced microbiome that keeps our bodies running smoothly. However, they can be disrupted by a range of factors, including poor diet, stress or taking a course of antibiotics.

Probiotics are the term we use to refer to the "good" bacteria that live in our bodies and help maintain good health.

They can even affect our mood, anxiety and depression.

We are each a "home" to roughly 39 trillion of these bacteria, (not sure who counted) and they help to expel "bad" bacteria, break-down fibre, and produce important vitamins like B12 and K2.

They weigh about 2 Kg (our brain only weighs 1.4 Kg!).

Up to 70% of our immune response mechanisms are resident in our gut, which is why maintaining our gastrointestinal health is essential.

A 2020 study entitled ***The gut microbiota and its interactions with cardiovascular disease*** [18] was undertaken to understand the connection between increased risk of CVD and gut bacteria.

They noted that;

---

[18] https://stamjournals.onlinelibrary.wiley.com/doi/full/10.1111/1751-7915.13524

"A growing body of literature supports the presence of interactions between the gut microbiota and hypertension."

and that ....

"Data from human and animals suggest that shifts in the gut microbiota play a fundamental role in diabetes, which is an important risk factor for CVD."

and also that......

"Lactobacillus rhamnosus GR-1 administration reduced infarct sizes and improved cardiac functions."

before ending with......

"Modulation of the gut microbiota via dietary intervention is a powerful approach for CVD prevention and therapy."

Diversity of bacteria as well as the volume is really important for robust health.

As a 2013 scholarly article[19] on bacteria states;

"In macro-ecosystems, several aspects of diversity are critical for conferring resilience, and the same features are likely important in microbial ecosystems including the human gut microbiota."

19

https://www.ncbi.nlm.nih.gov/pmc/articles/PMC3577372/?refcod
e=vpm_go&campaign=2038903639&keyword=&gclid=CjwKCAiAg
8OBBhA8EiwAlKw3kkNDo95bco08n0r7bCTFrieI76kBKu57y_x1u
A8_sUyOQc5mJ37wRRoCnEsQAvD_BwE

We are rapidly uncovering how the health and diversity of our gut microbiome is the source of our overall health.

We need gut microbes for:

- A robust immune system
- Neurocognitive development
- Balanced mood and behaviour
- Healthy hormonal functions

In fact, so many of our chemical and physiological responses come directly from the gut, that it is often referred to in medical circles as the 2nd brain, and there are a wealth of resources describing how a balanced and flourishing gut bacteria is the core of robust health.

We have something called an Enteric Nervous System (ENS).

The ENS from the gastrointestinal tract, is in constant communication with the brain via the vagus nerve, and it's now becoming clear that all those signals flowing back and forth can influence our decisions, mood and general well-being.

The ENS is awash with neurotransmitters, the biochemicals that are vital to brain activity. Evidence is emerging that the ENS even plays a role in depression.

For example, around 95 per cent of the body's serotonin (the chemical that makes us feel happy and positive, and is lacking when depression occurs) is produced not by the brain, but by the ENS, and is affected by what we eat, the state of our microbiome and the signals sent along the vagus nerve to the brain.

So gut health is critical for many hormonal functions as well as having a massive impact on mental health, which as we have also covered in this book, has a huge impact on heart health.

We need lots of microbes for a healthy existence, and how clean we've become is a serious problem.

We need exposure to more bacteria in order to improve our gut bacteria balance, and even things like stroking animals help to expose us to greater bacteria that strengthen or microbiome.

Some of the advice in order to improve your gut health includes:

- Eat local, seasonal, high-fibre vegetables

- Don't clean your hands too much

- Eat fermented foods

- Eat a wide range of foods

- Drink a bit of alcohol (I like to adhere to this one particularly)

- Spend more time outside

- Avoid antibiotics!

Dave Asprey is a three-time New York Times bestselling science author, host of the Webby award-winning podcast Bulletproof Radio, and has been featured on the Today Show, CNN and in The New York Times.

After years living a terribly unhealthy lifestyle working in the IT industry as a senior executive for product development, overweight and depressed, Dave set-out on a journey to apply his considerable brainpower and understanding of "systems" to unravel the "code" behind human development and health, losing 100 pounds in the process.

In one of his books, *Game Changers* Dave explains.

"Spending time in nature nourishes your brain and your gut, helps your cells create more energy and is at least as effective at treating depression as pharmaceuticals."

"It is essential to make the time to do something so basic that many people make the mistake of overlooking.....going outside."

Dave's mission is to empower the world with information that unlocks the Super Human in everyone with improvements in sleep quality, energy, sexual performance and longevity.

He has a point regarding the great outdoors.

We evolved for generation after generation over thousands of years living in, and with, the grass, air, water, soil and microbiome.

Yet it is not only possible, but entirely likely, that many of us live our lives without walking on grass, breathing unfiltered clean air, drinking natural water or rolling in soil on any given day.

We live in a domesticated environment, surrounded by our domesticated pets and eat domesticated food adapted (genetically modified, agriculturally farmed) to be a certain size, shape and taste that we can replicate, package, transport and store more easily.

We are essentially a domestic sub-species of the humans we should be.

No wonder we are so weak and susceptible to injuries, disease and poor health and vitality.

We will pass this weakened DNA on to the next generation...which become weaker and more susceptible still. And so it goes on as we pass these weaknesses from generation to generation.

Now I know this is a fairly extreme view of where we are as a species right now, and it ignores the developments in brain function, science and civilisation, but it does help you to understand that our environments impact on us is damaging physiologically and it is getting worse.

In order for our children to be more robust, we must be more robust, and in order for us to be more robust we can do a lot worse than getting outside.

This afternoon I plan to head out windsurfing in a harbour that is packed full of birds, and where the murky water I wade out into is silt-ridden from the flow of the river Stour, and salty from the incoming tide into Christchurch.

The hundreds of swans that call it their home, along with seagulls, terns and ducks have probably all been "crapping" in the water all morning.

It will look and taste foul....but I will no doubt fall in and be completely submerged a number of times attempting the near impossible feat (for me at least) of a fast-tack on my board.

As I chuckle a bit to myself after spitting-out the salty, dirty slush that fills my mouth in these moments, I know I will be healthier as a consequence.

A hot shower and a cuppa awaits....and when I sit looking out at the water, however cold, tiring, dirty and wet it gets I am *always* glad I went out.

I feel warm, relaxed, happy and grateful.

Want great brain health, and great heart health?

Get Dirty!

Keep your gut bacteria healthy:

- Eat foods with good levels of digestible fibre

- Consider probiotic supplementation

- Reduce stress, which can affect our microbiome

If you want to take probiotic supplements, those that contain at least 1 billion colony forming units, and containing the genus Lactobacillus, Bifidobacterium or Saccharomyces boulardii seem to be recommended.

It is advisable to perform your own research if you have specific conditions that may be helped by good bacteria. Each genus (type) of bacteria encompasses numerous strains that produce different results, so you may be low on a specific type of bacteria which is aggravating your condition.

Environment

I have outlined the effect of environmental toxins as a catalyst for inflammation and oxidation in the section on What Causes Heart Attacks.

We can try to limit our exposure to the leading environmental toxins by limiting our exposure to:

- Polluted air
- Cigarette smoke
- Vegetable Oils
- Heavily processed foods
- Fossil fuels
- Lead
- Old paint
- Chemical fertilisers
- Household mould

When choosing what to eat, where to live, how to heat your home, it is worth sparing a thought for the toxins you are exposing yourself to, and mitigate them as much as you can.

Supplements

Nan's Chapter Summary: Supplements can be a great way to improve the quantities of certain nutrients that can work to improve genetic issues that we may have discovered we suffer from.

Sometimes very high doses of certain vitamins and minerals can be needed to create a more dramatic effect in somebody that is deficient, or who suffers from heart disease.

Vitamin C and vitamin D are great examples where supplementing with much more than the recommended daily allowance (RDA)can have very beneficial effects on preventing heart disease.

The section towards the end of the book explains the benefits of taking supplements and how they can be used as a treatment.

Supplements are defined as **anything that we consume that contains a dietary ingredient.**

Dietary ingredients include vitamins, minerals, amino acids, and herbs or botanicals, as well as other substances that can be used to **supplement** our diet.

Medicine is defined as **a drug or other preparation for the treatment or prevention of disease.**

I find that it is often hard to define the difference between the two, except that generally I think of supplements as less processed, more natural and part of a general eating pattern, and medicine or drugs as more likely to be a man-made combination of chemicals to treat a specific illness or symptom for a short period of time.

Do we need to take supplements prevent heart disease? No, not always.

If we have no significant development of atherosclerosis, aren't from a genetically compromised group with an inherited risk-factor and eat nutrient-dense, minimally processed foods which enrich our bodies then there is generally no specific requirement for supplementation.

Often, though, we choose a sub-optimal diet, which over time can lead to deficiencies in certain nutrients which can increase risk. If this is the case, supplementation can get us back to a level of optimal vitamin and mineral balance.

Additionally, some of us have genetic heart disease risk-factors which may be modified or reduced by supplementation.

Personally, my philosophy is to treat any physical challenge or illness I face in the most natural way possible.

I start by eating better quality food, sleeping more, drinking more water, focussing on exercise and getting plenty of fresh air and sunlight exposure.

If these things don't start to cure me, then I might research the problem to understand more about the causes, and then see if there are any natural remedies, supplements or therapies that might help.

Lastly, if all of these things have failed I might go to a doctor and see if there is some reason that I may need a medical treatment.

For some of us heart disease is created or exacerbated by genetic factors that may be particularly challenging to discover, or treat.

These people may be clear candidates for some form of medical intervention, either to understand the exact cause, or to highlight any dietary or genetic idiosyncrasies that might be an underlying cause of heart disease.

However, this is rare, and the vast majority, and by that I mean pretty much all of us, can prevent or reverse heart disease with lifestyle interventions and the right mix of diet and supplements to overcome our genetic challenges, or at least reduce their impact.

Let me give you one great example.

Linus Pauling was an American chemist, biochemist, chemical engineer, peace activist, author, and educator.

He published more than 1,200 papers and books, of which about 850 dealt with scientific topics. *New Scientist* called him *one of the 20 greatest scientists of all time*, and he was rated the 16th most important scientist in history in 2000.

For his scientific work, Pauling was awarded the Nobel Prize in Chemistry in 1954. For his peace activism, he was awarded the Nobel Peace Prize in 1962.

He is one of four individuals to have won more than one Nobel Prize (the others being Marie Curie, John Bardeen and Frederick Sanger). Of these, he is the only person to have been awarded two unshared Nobel Prizes, and one of two people to be awarded Nobel Prizes in different fields, the other being Marie Curie.

Pauling was one of the founders of the fields of quantum chemistry and molecular biology.

You get the idea, Linus Pauling was a brilliant man.

In 1973, he founded what is now the Linus Pauling Institute of Science and Medicine.

He directed research on vitamin C, became especially interested in the possible role of vitamin C in preventing atherosclerosis, and published three case reports on the use of lysine and vitamin C to relieve angina.

During the 1990s, Pauling put forward a comprehensive plan for the treatment of heart disease using lysine (an amino acid) and vitamin C, referred to as Pauling Therapy.

Proponents of Pauling Therapy believe that heart disease can be treated and even cured using lysine and Vitamin C.

In 1989, Matthias Rath began working at the Linus Pauling Institute of Science and Medicine.

Rath had come from Germany, where he and his colleagues had uncovered evidence that the cause of plaque development in atherosclerosis (the hardening of arteries brought about by cholesterol deposits) was NOT a direct result of the presence of Low Density Lipoprotein (LDL).

Rath and Pauling worked together until Pauling died, but between them they have uncovered some interesting facts around heart disease, scurvy (yes really), collagen and vitamin C.

Scurvy, a condition that seems to only exist in films of doomed ship voyages in the 13th century, is a disease resulting from a lack of vitamin C (ascorbic acid).

In the 13th century, the Crusaders frequently suffered from scurvy.

In the 1497 expedition of Vasco da Gama, the curative effects of citrus fruit were already known for treating this condition.

Early symptoms of scurvy included weakness, feeling tired and sore arms and legs.

Without treatment, decreased red blood cells, gum disease, changes to hair, and bleeding from the skin would occur.

As scurvy worsened, poor wound healing and personality changes would precede death from infection or bleeding.

Why is this relevant?

Recently scurvy has made a bit of a comeback, as our modern diets contain less and less vitamin C.

Our artery walls are made robust and smooth by collagen, which is produced with vitamin C, so when we are low on vitamin C (in a pre-scurvy state) one of the first impacts of depleted collagen is weakened and cracking artery walls, the inflammation of which (through oxidised LDL) are the initiators of atherosclerosis.

In his book *Why Animals Don't Get Heart Attacks But Humans Do!* Matthius Rath MD explains;

"All animals, with only a few exceptions, produce large quantities of vitamin C in their bodies (2- 20 grams /day) to support optimum collagen production necessary for maintaining healthy and elastic blood vessels."

As I have mentioned previously, humans can no longer produce vitamin C, although most other mammals can.

"Animals don't get heart attacks because they produce large amounts of vitamin C, which optimises the production of collagen and other reinforcement molecules, stabilising the walls of the arteries and preventing atherosclerotic deposits."

"This is why animals do not die of heart attacks, even if some of them, such as bears, have very high blood cholesterol levels (600 mg/dl)."

Hmmmm….bears…..they have 3 times the concentration of cholesterol as a human, but no heart disease!

This is where it makes sense for you to Use Your Head to Heal Your Heart. Clearly it doesn't make any sense that cholesterol causes heart disease with this information. But I have rammed that point home hard enough.

Back to Dr Rath.

"In contrast , humans have lost the ability of vitamin C production and its daily dietary intake is often insufficient to assure optimum vascular health."

One of the many scientific references [20] in Rath's book, explains the effect when analysing artery walls of mice (which had been genetically modified so that like humans they did not produce their own vitamin C).

Given adequate or inadequate levels of vitamin C;

"The most striking effects of the marginal dietary vitamin C were alterations in the wall of aorta, evidenced by the disruption of elastic laminae, smooth muscle cell proliferation, and focal endothelial desquamation of the luminal surface. Thus, marginal vitamin C deficiency affects the vascular integrity."

In other words, the mice with less vitamin C had weakened and vulnerable artery walls.

A study [21] published in the **American Heart Journal** in 2011 examined the association between vitamin C concentrations and heart failure in 9,187 men and 11,112 women aged between 39 and 79 years old.

The researchers found that the risk of heart failure occurring was reduced when higher levels of vitamin C were present.

Conversely, people with the lowest levels of vitamin C had the highest risk of developing the condition.

Rath and Pauling discovered that LP(a) (the molecule that most highly predicts heart attack risk and which 20% of us genetically produce

---

[20]   https://pubmed.ncbi.nlm.nih.gov/10639167/

[21]   https://www.dr-rath-foundation.org/2018/04/scientific-research-confirms-micronutrients-prevent-heart-failure/

in dangerously high quantities) becomes less "sticky" and is then less able to accelerate atherosclerosis, when it becomes "coated" with two amino acids, proline and lysine.

Proline is an important amino acid which, like vitamin C, plays a role in collagen production.

You can pack in a healthy dose of proline by enjoying foods like asparagus, mushrooms, cabbage, bell peppers, strawberries and broccoli.

Lysine cannot be synthesised by humans, but instead is one of the essential amino acids which must be obtained from the diet.

Lysine plays several roles in humans, including the cross-linking of collagen polypeptides.

Lysine is mainly found in high amounts in meat, fish and dairy.

So, here we have two distinguished scientists, who dedicated many years of research into heart disease, and discovered simple supplemental remedies can have a massive effect on the prevention or reversal of heart disease.

Why is it then, that when esteemed scientists studies, and trials in humans, demonstrate that simple supplementation with pretty inexpensive vitamins and amino acids can dramatically improve the health of a high proportion of the population, (at highest risk of heart disease) that no doctor would think to mention it to a patient?

Does this have something to do with the fact that there is no patent on vitamin C, but over \$1 Trillon per year is made selling statins through patented brand names like Atorvastatin or Lovastatin?

Is it because doctors are paid bonuses to prescribe drugs, but are not paid to recommend supplements?

Possibly.

Is it because funding for research comes from the food and pharmaceutical companies, whose vested interests is in keeping us medicated, and which creates a negative cycle where medical experts that don't produce the right conclusions either don't get research funding, or have their results "buried"?

This has certainly been an issue in the past.

Is it because Big Pharma and Big Agriculture and Big Sugar (the terms for the most powerful companies in these sectors), companies like Coca Cola, Kelloggs, Pfizer, Merck, AstraZeneca, etc lobby governments and influence government health guidelines (despite the research showing that *their* foods make us sick) and then we are prescribed a "life sentence" of *their* drugs which may have little positive effects, but many damaging ones?

Absolutely, without question!

Is it because the medical training curriculum, which results in the qualifications to enable doctors to practice medicine, has a foundation based on biased research funded by the businesses mentioned above?

Yes!....100%.

I strongly believe we should look to supplements before we look to medicate.

Statins are one of the most prescribed medications in the world. They are undoubtedly the most mis-prescribed drug in the world.

There were 71 million statin prescription items dispensed in the UK alone in 2018.

In a recent paper by Stephanie Seneff BS, MS, EE, PhD (yes she really has earned all of these graduation acronyms) from the Massachusetts Institute of Technology, called ***How Statins Really Work Explains Why They Don't Really Work*** she articulates that statins cause more harm than good;

"The impact of the damage due to the statin anti-cholesterol mythology extends far beyond those who actually consume the statin pills."

"Cholesterol has been demonised by the statin industry, and as a consequence Americans have become conditioned to avoid all foods containing cholesterol. This is a grave mistake, as it places a much bigger burden on the body to synthesize sufficient cholesterol to support the body's needs, and it deprives us of several essential nutrients."

"Cholesterol is a remarkable substance, without which all of us would die".

"Statins slowly erode the muscle cells over time. After several years have passed, the muscles reach a point where they can no longer keep up with essentially running a marathon day in and day out. The muscles start literally falling apart, and the debris ends up in the kidney, where it can lead to rhabdomyolysis, which is often fatal."

She continued;

"31 of our statin reviews contained references to "rhabdomyolysis" as opposed to none in the comparison set. Kidney failure, a frequent consequence of rhabdomyolysis, showed up 26 times among the statin reviews."

Seneff is one of many leading minds that have analysed the scientific data and have become so shocked at the lack of efficacy, and the terrible side effects, of statins that she has dedicated much of her recent life to exposing the dangers of taking statins.

Dr Duane Graveline is another. In his book **The Dark Side Of Statins And The Wonder of Cholesterol** he summarised the current position from the scientific community relating to statins:

"After extensive review of all available studies relating to the cholesterol lowering benefits of statin drugs, scientists pulled the rug out from under the government sanctioned cholesterol levels for reducing cardiovascular disease. Their conclusion: "Current clinical evidence does not demonstrate that therapy to achieve proposed low LDL cholesterol levels is beneficial or safe."

This was announced in 2006. We are now in 2021.

Has this conclusion reached your doctor yet? My guess based on my experience is that it hasn't.

We know statins are extremely harmful, and have very poor efficacy in treating heart disease. But they make a lot of money for some of the largest companies on the planet, and reward doctors financially when prescribing them.

We know supplements like vitamin C can have a massive positive health impact. But they make no money for pharmaceutical companies and no doctors are rewarded financially for advising their use.

Later in the book, I will explain the role of some of the key supplements that might help to improve your susceptibility to heart disease, and when and how to take them.

Anti-Oxidants and Dietary Hacks

We often read or hear that certain foods, herbs or spices are "heart healthy" and in many cases they are.

Turmeric is a great example.

I have often seen turmeric attributed to great heart health, along with other items like resveratrol, pomegranates, grapefruits, blueberries, dark chocolate, beetroot, etc.

These individual foods and herbs often tend to have either anti-oxidant qualities (which combat oxidative stress) or stimulate a positive processes in the body, such as increased nitric oxide production (which dilates the blood vessels) or something similar.

Here is an example of how this can work.

Adiponectin is a hormone created by fat cells and is used to regulate metabolic processes, such as how the body uses fat for energy.

High blood levels of adiponectin are associated with a reduced risk of heart attacks.

Low levels of adiponectin are more likely to be found in people who are obese, and those with lower levels are at increased risk of heart attacks.

Interestingly adiponectin levels can be increased by eating fats (particularly avocados it seems) and also from consuming turmeric, red wine and coffee.

Understanding that certain foods support the increase of such a positive contributor to your heart health is useful to know.

There are many nutritionists, researchers, medical experts and functional medicine practitioners that provide great information about substances like these and how they can benefit good health.

Often they create blogs, and links to research, and can be found online.

Always be conscious of evaluating new information with a critical eye.

NB. Whenever coffee is mentioned as a health-positive anti-oxidant, I hope it is clear that this means organic coffee, least roasted and not instant coffee!......OK!....just checking!

Positivity and Thoughts

Nan's Chapter Summary: *Our thoughts are things that we consume, and they can have a positive or negative impact on our hormone balance.*

The previous section on depression and anxiety touched on how our mental health can play a role in creating a hormone imbalance, and that can affect our blood pressure and our management of blood sugar as well as our gut bacteria.

We should work to create and environment that encourages relaxation and allows ourselves to de-stress, and we should encourage positive relationships and discourage negative relationships where we can to ensure that our thoughts remain as positive as possible to maintain good heart health.

How do we consume thoughts?

If one of the negative consequences of eating a diet that elevates blood glucose is hormone imbalance that can accelerate heart disease, then surely anything that we take-in which alters our hormone balance negatively might also be considered unwanted consumption.

Like the food that we accept into our stomachs, the thoughts, concepts, opinions and beliefs that we accept into our minds can have a profound effect on our hormonal balance, and therefore our physical health, as well as developing into long-term mental health challenges.

Mindhealth 360[22] reports that;

---

22   https://www.mindhealth360.com/contributor/negative-thought-patterns-and-beliefs/

"Repeated negative thoughts, such as anger, resentment, fear, or depression, cause our bodies to release the stress hormones cortisol and adrenaline."

For example, if we hear a rumour that our company is down-sizing and making staff redundant, we may have thoughts about how this might impact us.

We might believe a really negative scenario about the future based on some assumptions about what might happen, we may dwell on this, we may procrastinate over how to respond, we may then experience fear for our financial security, anxiety about how that may affect our relationships, worry about all the people we are responsible for.

All of this leads to chronic stress, for which we pay a terrible price hormonally.

And in the scenario above this might last for months, affecting our sleep, making us feel depressed and lethargic, leading to increased cortisol, which stimulates insulin and which in-turn leads us to drink more alcohol and eat more "comfort" food.

Before ever having received the bad news that our worst fears have been realised, we have created significant damage to ourselves physically.

You may recognise this in yourself, or in others.

It is hard to watch somebody that you care about causing themselves so much pain as well as physical and mental damage, from negative thoughts.

Ordinarily cortisol, the key stress hormone, peaks in the blood in the morning and decreases throughout the day.

However, in about half of people that suffer with depression, it peaks earlier and does not level-off or decrease in the same way.

To make matters worse, some of the symptoms of depression, such as low energy and lack of motivation, can make getting regular exercise, eating healthy foods, and sticking to a relaxation protocol very difficult.

The key to resolving this is to break the cycle and shift the body away from this chronic stress response towards a relaxation response.

When this happens our cortisol levels drop and our self-repair mechanisms get back to work.

Depression and cortisol seem to work in lock-step.

If we improve one, we improve the other.

When surveyed in June 2020, almost one in five UK adults (19.2%) were likely to be experiencing some form of depression.

Here are a few ways we can lower our cortisol levels, and start to work towards breaking the cycle of anxiety and depression:

- **Eat a low-glycemic diet.** Sugar (and elevated blood glucose from carbohydrates and heavily processed foods) can increase adrenaline and cortisol. Consume plenty of saturated fats, proteins and greens to help regulate cortisol and insulin.

- **Engage in regular physical activity.** Moderate physical exercise does wonders to relieve stress and lower cortisol levels. High-Intensity Interval Training is also fantastic for managing stress and insulin. Go for a walk, or perform some sprints.

- **Practice meditation.** Even a few minutes of meditation a day has a cumulative, positive effect on your stress levels. A 15 minute meditation session each morning will help start the day in a calm and relaxed state.

- **Get proper rest.** Insomnia causes high cortisol for up to 24 hours. Interruptions to sleep, even if brief, can also increase our levels and disrupt daily hormone patterns. Try to get to bed at the same time every night and wake up at the same time each morning. Try not to eat, drink alcohol or engage in screen-time for a few hours before bedtime, and sleep in a cool room.

- **Be sociable.** Even if we sometimes feel like some solitary time, reaching-out my to others and regularly engaging with friends and family is very important. Isolation and loneliness increase stress, anxiety, and depression. It's important to find ways to connect socially with other people to manage stress.

- **Laugh.** Researchers have found that laughing significantly reduces stress hormone levels. In one study in Korea[23], 8 weeks of laughter therapy (sign me up for that course) decreased the cortisol levels of student nurses, and improved their psychological wellbeing. So the next time you're feeling anxious, try watching a comedy.

Of course this doesn't resolve some of the real world issues that may be catalysts for anxiety or depression, such as relationship issues, money worries, bereavement, and a many other life challenges, but these strategies should form part of the bedrock of good mental health.

If you do have additional worries, please speak with somebody.

The **Stress Management Society** have lots of information and resources to help deal with stress, and can be found at www.stress.org.uk

---

[23]   https://www.ncbi.nlm.nih.gov/pmc/articles/PMC7045881/

If you don't have anybody that you feel able to speak with, Samaritans offers a free, 24 hour, confidential telephone listening service on 116 123.

RECUPERATION

The **R** in C.R.A.S.H. is Recuperation.

Recuperation is a global term that I am using to mean rest, recovery, relaxation and basically **taking-it-easy** for a while.

Our bodies, and our hearts, minds and muscles….**and our cars** all have something in common.

If we **over**-use them they become weaker, tired and start to fail.

If we **under**-use them they also become weaker (or atrophy, which is the medical term used to describe "wasting-away").

What enables these parts of our body to thrive, grow strong and repair are three things:

1.   Stress

2.   Positive Post-Stress Environment Factors

3.   Rest

Stress comes in many forms:

-   **Emotional stress** - sadness, grief, anxiety, depression

-   **Physical stress** - obesity, climbing mountains

-   **Work stress** - low control - high demand

-   **Pharmacological stress** - drugs, alcohol, medications, etc

-   **Infective stress** - flu, pneumonia, tooth-extraction stress

Think about our muscles. They don't grow without exercise. Exercise is the first element, the "stress" that we put our muscles under.

277

Too little stress and they won't grow, and they will atrophy.

Too much stress and they will tear, or take a long time to recover and we will become weaker.

But the right amount of stress and they will be stimulated to improve in strength to meet the demands that we are placing on them, *but only if they also have the proteins and amino acids in our body to repair and grow*, this is the second element.

They need an environment with the right nutrition. Protein shakes, chicken, eggs, meat…. the right diet containing enough of the essential amino acids.

Lastly, they need a period of rest, where the nutrition we have consumed helps muscle fibres to grow and develop ready for the next period of stress.

This is the *Recuperation.*

If any of these elements is missing, or sub-optimal, our muscles will not grow stronger.

The same is true of our brain.

We can stress our brain by reading, learning a new language or musical instrument or skill that requires co-ordination, and it will form new neural pathways and grow.

We notice we improve at what we are learning, but only if we get a chance to rest afterwards, relax our minds, and have a peaceful environment and good sleep.

If these elements of recuperation don't accompany the stress, and all we do is force ourselves to study harder, and harder, then we will start to feel overwhelmed, forgetful and anxious which will make learning impossible and our memory and mental health will suffer.

How much stress, how much rest and what environmental factors work best for us is often a function of our unique, individual characteristics, from genetic make-up to personality type, age and sex and learning style so we each need to find the right balance that works for us.

Some people lift heavy weights and grow strong but need a week-off afterwards to rest in-between gym sessions, whilst others can train every other day and recover well.

Everybody is different. But the principle is the same.

At certain times we can feel better able to handle stressors.

For example, it is counter-productive and futile to expect go to the gym and have a fantastic intense workout if we were up all night with a crying new-born child, or are dealing with stressful challenges at work, or are feeling upset about a relationship issue for example.

But when we are rested and fresh and full of energy without other stressors, we can put your foot on the gas and train hard.

By all means take advice relating to health and fitness from those that you trust, and that have credibility, and a proven track-record. But in the end you will need to work out what works for *YOU* and learn to adapt routines that suit *YOU!*

Similarly our hearts need to be exercised and rested, stressed and then provided a period of recuperation. After all, it is the most important muscle in the body.

So here are the main areas of Recuperation in the C.R.A.S.H. model, and how they affect heart health.

Sleep

Nan's Chapter Summary: Our hormones become unbalanced, and we are more likely to be stressed, hungry and unhappy as a consequence of poor sleep.

It is a key foundation of good health to sleep deeply, and with as few interruptions as possible, throughout the night.

Creating an evening routine that encourages less mental activity, natural light, less alcohol, and a moderate temperature can really help to gradually improve the quality of sleep for those that have issues in this area.

If you are anything like me, you will think back to childhood days and remember being able to go to bed and fall asleep within minutes of your head hitting the pillow.

Nowadays, I can take anything from 20 minutes to 2 or 3 hours to get off to sleep, will often wake in the night restless, may also wake up to go to the toilet (its an age thing!) and will wake up sometimes worried about missing the morning alarm on my phone (how dumb is that!).

It is common for me to get less than 6 hours of badly interrupted, restless sleep.

This is incredibly bad for heart-health for a number of reasons.

Sleep is a time that our bodies perform repair functions, as well as providing much of the rest that was mentioned in the introduction to Recuperation in the C.R.A.S.H. model.

If we sleep badly, this acts as a stressor much like an argument with a colleague at work. It can elevate cortisol and insulin and can leave us feeling tired and anxious when we wake-up.

Not a great way to start a new day.

Additionally, the hormones that send us reaching for high carbohydrate-laden foods, leptin and ghrelin are affected by sleep.

Sleepfoundation.org states that;

"Ghrelin stimulates appetite, whilst leptin decreases it. When the body is sleep-deprived, the level of ghrelin spikes, while the level of leptin falls, leading to an increase in hunger."

If we do not sleep well, we will wake-up hungry and tired.

You know the routine.

We are startled-awake by our alarm clock and rush out of the door, toast-in-hand ......and so start the roller-coaster of hormonal disruption that exacerbates feelings of stress.

Maybe our day is a little less hectic and disorganised than that...but it is common to start the day with cereal or toast, and have woken at a time not dictated by our circadian rhythm, so the effect is essentially the same, but maybe a little less obvious.

This type of start to the day elevates stress hormones that when consistently and chronically elevated will harm our health in every way imaginable.

Additionally, it has been shown that not having good sleep will mean we start our day more resistant to insulin than if we slept well, even before the poor food choices that we are about to make.

In the *Impact of sleep debt on metabolic and endocrine function* a 1999 study[24] published in *The Lancet* it was shown that

---

24

https://www.sciencedirect.com/science/article/abs/pii/S01406736
99013768

just one week of less, than optimal, sleep could result in 30% more insulin resistance.

Starting the day with a good morning routine helps us to manage the day better, so we would be advised to give ourselves the time to do what we need to in the morning, waking up without a rush, rested from the night before, and with a morning routine that maintains a calm, relaxed and prepared state.

If you want to meditate, get some yoga practice, make coffee, get dressed and be at the station in time for the train that gets you into work 15 minutes early, then plan around that realistically.

Set a gentle alarm with a snooze setting at a time that lets you ease yourself awake over a 15 minute period, so you don't need to rush.

Sounds like utopia for most of us, and there will be times in our lives when this is harder than others (like when we have a baby or small children to disrupt our patterns).

Being prepared and planning a routine though, is key to starting to sleep better, and when we sleep better, everything else is more manageable.

At the other end of the day, stress can prevent us from getting-off to sleep in the first place.

If we are worried about work, finances, our relationship or our health, we can find that our minds are too active to sleep or we may just be too distressed.

Just like a good morning routine, a good evening routine really helps us to get into a pattern that will gradually get us back into restful habits.

It is good to plan to "wind-down" well in advance of bedtime. If we make work or social calls in the evening and get embroiled in an argument, a difficult challenge, or vocalise our feelings of stress and anxiety (or our friends feelings of stress and anxiety) in a call, it may be something that creates stress or anxiety in us, that can be hard to un-wind from.

Many of us feel the need to constantly be available to our friends, family and work through emails and calls, at any time of the day and night.

If you are an ER doctor on-call, or have a friend that is in great distress that may need you, then of course it is understandable that you may have priorities that will disrupt your desire for a good nights sleep, but if not then maybe setting some telephonic boundaries is appropriate.

It is often thought to be a good practice to place our phones on Do Not Disturb as a priority (if appropriate for you) in the early evening, and minimise stimulants after 7pm. Whilst this is a difficult challenge for many (me included) it does really help to start to restore calm to evenings.

Many of us go to bed when we are over-tired, or force ourselves to stay up to finish watching a film. This is a particularly bad habit of mine.

If a new series (like Ozarks for example) comes onto Netflix, I seem incapable of watching an episode and heading off to bed at 10pm. I will look at my partner and pull the face that says "let's just watch one more….pleeeeease!" And then 3 episodes later will head off to bed at 1am.

It sometimes takes 2 or 3 days for me to recover from the tiredness, and I notice that I might make poorer choices with food, or skip exercise in the following few days.

In short, I compromise my routine and my health by bingeing on TV, instead of spreading out my Netflix doses throughout the week.

Daft really! Would it be better to spread the series out over 2 weeks and feel great? Of course it would. Will I do that when the next series is released? Probably not!

What can I say?…..I'm an idiot!

It is better to have a set time each night when we aim to be in bed and sleeping, not in bed doing other things, and try to keep to this time most evenings.

Presuming parties and nights-out are not a daily occurrence, this will help your body to start conforming to a pattern, and you will notice that you naturally start to feel tired at this time, after a while.

This works in the same way as waking…you will notice that when you get used to waking at a set time each day, you will often wake at that time even without an alarm clock. The body likes routine.

It seems good practice to set a time for dinner and regularly eat well before bedtime, so we don't feel bloated, and aren't digesting food when heading off to bed.

In an ideal world it is good to try to keep sleeping in-line with circadian rhythms, although this is not always practical.

A circadian rhythm is a natural, internal process that regulates the sleep-wake cycle and repeats on each rotation of the Earth, roughly every 24 hours.

I know this is very idealistic, as work times and social lives don't tend to fit-in with the orbiting of planets around the sun, but the closer we keep bedtime and waking to sunset and sunrise, the better our body responds and performs.

Of course with modern technology we have ways to mimic sunset and sunrise, like lighting, curtains, etc.

Bedrooms, and lounging environments, do seem to promote sleep better when the lighting is more subtle and mimics sunset, so bulbs that are more red in colour and lampshades that emit light upwards from a side table, rather than blue lightbulbs emitting downwards from the ceiling, are preferable.

On the subject of light, and its colour. There has been lots of re-search on devices that emit blue light, and the effect of blue light on sleep. I have not been able to find enough definitive evidence that blue light is an issue per-se though.

It has been hard to prove whether the blue light from a device dam-ages sleep, or the stimulation of the social media or book that was read from the device providing stimulus is the cause of disrupted sleep.

It is sometimes the case that reading a book is seen as a way to have ones eyes become more tired, and helps some people to sleep.

In general though stimulus is something that will disrupt sleep.

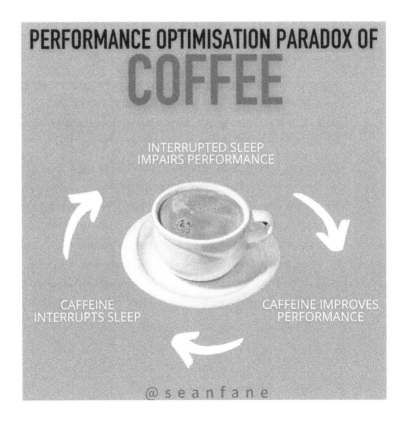

Caffeine (particularly in the form of coffee) is the most widely consumed stimulant in the world.

Coffee is a bit of a poisoned chalice for many of us.

While there is substantial evidence that caffeine enhances performance, caffeine withdrawal leads to deficits[25] in cognitive, emotional, and behavioural processes, as the 2018 article called ***Effects of caffeine on sleep quality and daytime functioning*** shows.

Also, whilst great to perk us up at 9am, coffee in the afternoon may disturb our sleep later that evening, so it is advisable to resist too much coffee after midday.

In order to get back to childlike levels of sleep quality and duration, and create hormonal balance, there are a number of top-tips which will help.

1. **Keep active during the day** - nothing helps more with sleep quality than feeling like you need it, and if you listen to your body, it will tell you to get some quality shut-eye if you have had an active day. Give-in to the urge when you feel it.

2. **Don't eat before bed** - Carbohydrates have the effect of making your body feel warm, and if you are carb-sensitive (as many are) can make you feel tired and drowsy, but much like alcohol, this should not be assumed to be sleep-promoting for a full evening. Eating too close to bedtime will stimulate the digestive process, increase blood glucose and elevate insulin (particularly if it is a high carbohydrate meal). All this activity does not make for prolonged, deep, restful sleep. Give yourself at least a cou-

---

ple of hours between your last meal and bed, and minimise carbohydrates and sugars in your last meal, and this will improve your sleep quality throughout the night.

3. **Have a boozy lunch** – OK, you don't *need* to have a boozy lunch, but if you are going to drink alcohol, you should know that it will affect your sleep negatively if it is still in your bloodstream when you head off to bed. Whilst it seems intuitive that alcohol would help you sleep by making you drowsy, like eating carbohydrates, the sugar in alcohol triggers insulin stimulation, and this along with giving your liver the task of "clearing" it out of your system actually damages your sleep quality. If you are going to have a glass of wine....have it with your lunch, not your dinner.

4. **Avoid water for 2 hours before bed** - this isn't a tip that everybody needs to follow, but if like me, your bladder seems to have shrunk to the size of an acorn, and you get up like clockwork at 4 am for a wee, then you aren't going to enjoy the benefits of full, rested, deep sleep. Being dehydrated is pretty bad for the heart, and drinking before bed if you are dehydrated is recommended as heart protective. Keep well hydrated throughout the day, then if you cut-out water an hour or two before bedtime, you can still go through the night with minimum sleep disruptions, and remain sufficiently hydrated, which would be preferable.

5. **Avoid caffeine after the morning** - The good decision to drink that morning cup of coffee that jolted you into life for a focussed day at the office, runs the risk of being a terrible decision later in the day, when it can affect your sleep, and make you very tired the next day. We can then get caught in a cycle of needing coffee again and repeat, slaves to the positive and negative consequences of the worlds most popular stimulant. Have

your last caffeine hit before 2pm (latest) to prevent it affecting your sleep.

6. **Scrap the screens** - Whether they are phones, computers, TV's of e-readers…..turn-off your blue-light-emitting devices a few hours before bed and don't allow them to disrupt your sleep. While light of any kind can suppress the secretion of melatonin, blue light at night does so more powerfully. Harvard researchers[26] and their colleagues conducted an experiment comparing the effects of 6.5 hours of exposure to blue light to exposure to green light of comparable brightness. The blue light suppressed melatonin for about twice as long as the green light and shifted circadian rhythms by twice as much (3 hours vs. 1.5 hours). There is, however, recent research[27] that refutes the theory that blue-light itself causes a reduction in sleep quality but does still concede that maybe the use of devices per-se causes sleep issues instead. Either way, brain stimulation at bedtime is a bad idea if you want to optimise sleep quality. If you need to use a screen right before bed, then maybe you could try using anti-blue light glasses to mitigate some of the potential for disruption.

7. **Night Light** - Whilst halogen ceiling lights look cool, and are very bright, their use all over a house can damage sleep-quality. In order to mimic the setting of the sun, and support your natural circadian rhythms, it has been shown to be very beneficial for your sleep-quality to use lower-level up-lighting (such as table lamps with shades) and red bulbs in the evening. Harvard

---

[26]   https://www.health.harvard.edu/staying-healthy/blue-light-has-a-dark-side

[27]   https://time.com/5752454/blue-light-sleep/

researchers suggest *"Use dim red lights for night lights. Red light is less likely to shift circadian rhythm and suppress melatonin."*

8. **Keep Cool** - Sleeping in a cool room[28] can help regulate your hormones and increase the production of melatonin, it has been suggested. Open a window or set the thermostat to go off at bedtime to keep your bedroom cool. Somewhere between 60F and 68F has been suggested as optimal.

Relaxation

Nan's Chapter Summary: *Relaxation is as important as exercise in keeping our body and mind healthy.*

Be sure to prioritise the things that help to calm you down, and relieve your stresses.

It's easy to tell someone to "Just relax" but much less easy to do.

Relaxation is such a broad term, but by this I mean the opposite of being in a constant state of stress or worry.

I say this as somebody that overthinks everything, and spends most of his time worrying if I have offended somebody by the way I worded a throw-away comment, or whether I have left it too long in between calls catching-up with my sister.

I also spend my time on flights imagining crash scenarios and how I might get out of the plane, and who I could save with me, or looking four cars ahead whilst driving anticipating whether a car will turn right

---

28 https://en.getmoona.com/blogs/mission-sleep/the-health-benefits-of-sleeping-at-cooler-temperatures

based on the head movements of the driver, before he has actually indicated.

Sound familiar? Maybe not, but if this is you, then know that all this constant worrying and over-thinking is not doing you any good. (Except if the plane you are on actually does crash, but you somehow manage to survive the impact.....a bit of a long-shot!)

The constant state of worry, or concern will raise your cortisol levels, in much the same way that I mentioned in the section on sleep, with the same negative long-term consequences.

Our lives are so busy and focussed, we want to achieve and be successful. We want to make the right decisions, but being relaxed doesn't mean never trying or not thinking things through. Just don't counter-productively dwell on thoughts, where you cannot know or control the outcome.

Besides all the negative aspects of dwelling on the past or worrying about the future, this behaviour also prevents you from enjoying your life right now, and that enjoyment can come from many different little things and make you feel positive, energised and grateful.

As Master Oogway said in Kung Fu Panda;

"Yesterday is history, tomorrow is a mystery, but today is a gift, which is why it is called the present!"

As a wise man once said, if you worry about a potential problem and then it happens, you end up dealing with it twice. Once when you anticipated it and once when it happened. One challenge, twice the stress.

Meditation, Mindfulness & Gratitude

Nan's Chapter Summary: *Mindfulness is the term that is used to describe living in the moment.*

When we fully engage with the people and the places in our lives we can feel more attached, and part of something. This creates feelings of well-being.

Gratitude, even for the little things, and even when you might think there isn't much to be grateful for, really helps top create a sense of peace and balance that removes stress and anxiety, and creates calm.

All of these little adjustments to how we look at life and engage with it, help to create a positive healthy hormone balance, and help us to cope with the challenges in life much better when they do come along.

Michael J Fox is a pretty inspirational chap.

Experiencing massive success early in his life as a teenage actor, he had money, fame and the world at his feet....and then he developed Parkinson's at the age of 29.

Within 9 years he was suffering quite badly from the symptoms, but had started to adjust to the mental challenge of accepting that his life was going to take a turn for the worse, but was determined to look for the good in every day.

These are a few quotes from him, which show the mentality that enabled him to cope, and then enjoy his life, despite the tumultuous change that he has gone through.

"Acceptance doesn't mean resignation; it means understanding that something is what it is and that there's got to be a way through it!"

"My happiness grows in direct proportion to my acceptance, and in inverse proportion to my expectations"

"Don't imagine the worst...if you imagine the worst and it happens, you've lived it twice!"

Meditation, mindfulness & gratitude are three very under-utilised, but extremely powerful healing and wellness practices.

Until my post-heart attack exploration of relaxation practice, the only people that I had encountered that had mentioned things like mindfulness and meditation were either friends going through a 'hippy-like' phase of emotional connection, or those that had tough mental health challenges that they were working through.

I certainly didn't know anybody that practiced these activities consciously or regularly as part of a strategy to maintain good health and balance.

And yet the more I have learned, and the more I have practiced these things myself, I have come to believe them to be extremely valuable and important aspects of health.

I have felt more generally calm, better able to cope with unexpected challenges, less triggered by (or willing to engage in) arguments, and more able to "let-go" of past situations that had been playing-on-my-mind, since engaging in gratitude and meditation each day.

I have already explained how stress hormones affect health, and these are all initiated to some degree by these triggers.

Scientific evidence supports the positive effects of these relaxation practices on heart health.

In *The Role of Gratitude in Well-being in Asymptomatic Heart Failure Patients*[29] the following was noted after examining associations between gratitude, relaxation and inflammation in 186 men and women with stage B asymptomatic:

---

[29]   https://www.ncbi.nlm.nih.gov/pmc/articles/PMC4566460/

"In correlational analysis, gratitude was associated with better sleep, less depressed mood, less fatigue, and better self-efficacy to maintain cardiac function".

"Patients expressing more gratitude also had lower levels of inflammatory biomarkers."

"Gratitude and spiritual well-being are related to better mood and sleep, less fatigue, and more self-efficacy, and that gratitude fully or partially mediates the beneficial effects of spiritual well-being on these endpoints."

"Efforts to increase gratitude may be a treatment for improving well-being in heart-failure patients' lives and be of potential clinical value."

Here are some tips to create a more relaxed approach to life and minimise the day-to-day stress you experience.

1. **Practice Mindfulness** - Being "mindful" is a great way of being focussed on the here-and-now, and provides a relaxing boost. There are many ways to practice mindfulness, but it essentially teaches you to connect with everything around you consciously. I used to walk my dogs with headphones on listening to a podcast or two, whilst completely ignoring the pooches as they ran off across the fields near me and into the river that I had barely noticed. When I practiced mindfulness on a dog walk, I could smell the river-water in the air, hear the sounds of a few different types of birds, sensed the temperature in the air, felt the sun on my neck, and felt completely uplifted! It is hard to feel stressed after that.

2. **Trust Yourself** - Deal with a problem when it arises and trust that, if you can work out what to do to resolve it in advance, then you will do the same thing should it actually arise. The let-go! Don't think about it again. Avoid anticipating a negative event that may not happen..

3. **Practice Gratitude** - This is much more powerful than I had expected. From letting go of past relationship issues, work challenges, resentment towards people that have wronged you, to really truly appreciating what you have now, however little that might be. This really makes you feel grateful, appreciative and relaxed. It is easier said than done, but adding 5 minutes of gratitude practice to the end of each meditation session every morning, or before bed every night, really makes a massive difference to your health and helps you feel better able to cope with life and enjoy everything in it. Start by writing three things you are grateful for in a notepad by your bed every night.

4. **Practice Meditation** - 15 minutes, twice a day (upon waking and then mid afternoon) can have enormous benefits on your cortisol levels over time. Stress is the body's response to unforeseen adversities. Studies[30] of regular meditators revealed that they have lower cortisol level in their brains, amongst other benefits to wellbeing and mental health.

Yoga

Well this makes it into *R* in the C.R.A.S.H. Model ...but it also could have made it into *A* for Activity as well.

Yoga can mean different things to different people.

Some see it as an exercise, but for me exercises are more to improve either muscular strength or cardiovascular endurance, and whilst certain styles of yoga can certainly improve these, I don't believe it is the most optimal route to either of those goals.

---

[30] https://psycnet.apa.org/record/1975-28039-001

It *does* help with relaxation and wellness overall in a very impactful way though, by creating a balance within your body.

We spend much of our lives stuck in physical positions that our bodies weren't designed for, like sitting in a car, slumped on a sofa, typing on a keyboard or holding a phone.

We then sleep on a mattress with a pillow and start all over again.

Even when we exercise, it isn't generally very well-balanced for the whole body.

If you play a racket sport for example, it might provide a good cardio workout, but it will impact one side of your body more than the other with a recurring movement unnatural to the body. Unless a programme of careful stretching and overall body exercise is maintained alongside your sport, it may take its toll on your body over time, and injuries, imbalances and accompanying physical discomfort can then arise.

Just go to any tennis club and look at all the players over 40 with a neoprene knee or elbow strap on, and you will get the picture.

Believe me, when you get to your 40's and upwards, your life can become a never-ending round of tennis elbow, rotator-cuff injuries, back problems, stiff neck, plantar fasciitis, shin-splints, etc.

I once heard a fellow tennis player joke that his clubs team was sponsored by Nurofen....and he was only half joking!

Yoga can help to eradicate these imbalances, and create flexibility and joint health, and comes in many forms now.

Some is faster-paced with more dynamic poses, and can be very challenging from a strength and flexibility point of view, but classic yoga to me is really beneficial for its unique ability to re-set the body, to prevent injuries and optimise our body's functional adaptation to life and sport.

It's funny, but even with a name like _downward dog_ describing a yoga pose, we seem to forget that even animals stretch to prepare themselves for each day, despite the fact that they don't abuse their bodies natural functional patterns quite as badly as we humans do, or sit in chairs.

Sauna

Nan's Chapter Summary: *If you have access to a sauna, it can reduce stress, and improve blood sugar levels, as well as reduce blood pressure.*

If you are in recovery for a heart attack, or are in the advanced stages of heart disease, then extremes of temperature will put your heart under increased stress, and this can be dangerous.

If, however, you have received confirmation from your doctor that it is safe for you to gradually introduce heat treatment as a therapy, it has some very positive outcomes.

Why is the sauna so good for us!?

I spent years hating the thought of even stepping into a sauna, and the heat felt so oppressive to me.

Asked if I would like to go into the sauna by friends at a health club, I would always politely decline the invitation.

Since my heart attack I have read a lot about heat and cold therapies, and sauna has jumped right up to the top of my recommendations for regular indulgence.

It seems, the heat from a sauna is good for much more than just healing tired muscles too.

According to Christian Assad M.D…

"There is tonnes of research in the use of sauna, medi-tation, adequate sleep as key in reversing insulin resistance. Many of us are stressed and we don't sleep well. Once you start looking at it and you get a birds-eye view, we can see that there are many different interventions from lifestyle that can impact the five variables of "metabolic syndrome" ...we can go with fasting, low-carb ketogenic, we can go with ade-quate sleep or episodes of HITT, sauna and meditation."

Ivor Cummins - The Fat Emperor Podcast, has this to say about saunas

"Sauna targets everything from insulin resistance, blood pressure, inflammation...research from Japan and Finland is very hard to ignore."

The reality is, heat treatment and also cold-therapy both instigate a stress response on the body, and the body adapts by waking itself-up from the slumber of normal life and kicks itself into gear.

It is often debated why heat and cold treatment are so effective at improving immune system function, reducing blood pressure, improving insulin sensitivity, improving mood and mental chemical balance.

The medical community is still in debate about the exact processes. Often during exposure to extremes of temperature, the stress response encourages the body to adapt favourably, accelerating hormonal changes, and then relaxing afterwards.

Research [31] in the ***Canadian Journal of Diabetes*** found that 20 minute infra-red sauna use, 3 times per week for three months, improved CVD risk factors, and improved insulin sensitivity.

"Infrared saunas are beneficial for the treatment of congestive heart failure, hypertension and obesity. As such, they may have a beneficial effect on cardiovascular (CV) health in those with type 2 diabetes."

The adaptation between heat and cold seems optimally favourable, so maybe the Finns and Swedes were onto something after all, with 2 minutes in a sauna swiftly followed by a dunk in an ice-cold plunge-pool, or a roll in the snow.

Whilst I know this hasn't answered the question of why a sauna is so good for our health, the overwhelming evidence is that it is, whether the mechanisms for this are fully understood or not.

---

[31] https://www.canadianjournalofdiabetes.com/article/S1499-2671(10)42007-9/abstract

ACTIVITY

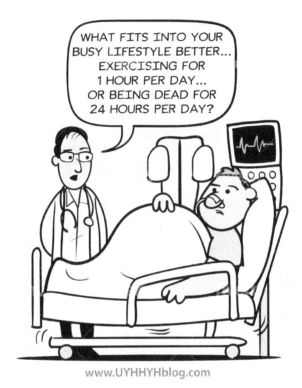

www.UYHHYHblog.com

The **A** in C.R.A.S.H. is Activity.

It will be no great surprise to you, I am sure, to discover that being active is good for your heart.

It has long been known that "keeping fit" through cardiovascular exercise (running, jogging, etc) keeps the heart strong and helps prevent heart disease.

There is an easy pitfall in this over-simplistic way of thinking though, so it is useful to explain how certain activities that you undertake can help protect your heart, because it's not all about going for a run.

N.E.A.T.

Nan's Chapter Summary: NEAT *is just a term for regular activity during the day. If you potter around in the garden, that is classed as NEAT. If you do the washing-up, that is classed as NEAT. Any activity that is not a specific sport or recognised physical endeavour will be classed as NEAT.*

The amazing thing is that people that are more generally active, and spend more time on their feet throughout the day, tend to actually generate better health than people that sit down most of the time and then do a burst of exercise in a gym, or play a sport.

If you are somebody that keeps your house and garden neat, then you probably have a high level of NEAT. Keep it up! It is really good for your heart-health.

N.E.A.T. is the catchy acronym for non-exercise activated thermogenesis.

This is a term used to describe the metabolic effect (essentially calories used) by just doing non-specific "stuff" ....like just moving, or "pottering" about the house.

Keeping active and using step-counters on phones and watches are examples of how we have collectively become more conscious of the power of NEAT.

Keeping active, keeping ones NEAT at a good level, is useful for a number of reasons, but it is particularly good for helping one improve insulin sensitivity.

It is also great for reducing blood-pressure.

Many of us spend most of our adult lives sitting at a desk, sitting on a sofa, sitting in a car and sitting to eat. Getting up and about very often….well….takes a "back-seat".

Having a generally active life, should be a fundamental requirement for everybody, because in the same way that a car sitting unused in a driveway for long periods of time will function poorly, your body will too if you don't keep it moving.

The term "use it or lose it!" has a lot of validity.

Very often we spend a short amount of time exercising, and then presume we have done enough to justify all of the remaining hours of the day we spend sitting in a car, on a train, on a sofa, at a desk or at a dinner table.

This is certainly not the best way to improve your overall health, and often when we work-up a sweat once a day exercising, or playing sport, we probably over-estimate the benefits somewhat.

In *The **Body Project*** [32] blog, health and lifestyle coach Melody Coleman articulates the relative benefits of being generally active, compared with having a desk job and working out once a day.

Coleman explains;

"A 13 year study on over 120,000 individuals published in the American Journal of Epidemiology found that inactive people who sat for more than 6 hours per day were up to 94% more likely to die during the study period than active people who sat for less than 3 hours per day. Shocking, right!?"

---

[32]   https://bodyprojectpt.com/blog/sedentary-lifestyle/

"I'm sorry to say this, but 2-3 hours spent exercising out of a total of 168 each week won't negate you having been sedentary for the best part of your 40+ hour working week."

Being active can involve getting the benefits of exercise, whilst not really feeling like you have needed to exercise, which for those that don't like running or the gym, is a good thing.

Whether it is going for a dog walk, gardening, cycling to the shops instead of driving, taking the stairs instead of the elevator, cleaning the house…all these have positive implications for health.

Anything that you do that makes you more active is like exercise for the body, and creates a very positive impact on your metabolism, and your hormone balance.

Coleman continues with a warning;

"If you continue to keep a sedentary lifestyle, then you will end up looking and feeling older than your years, suffer from more serious health issues, and end up immobile in old age, confined to your chair. You'll also die sooner. It's a harsh truth, but understanding it opens up a world of opportunities for us. With this knowledge we are guided to make much better choices about how we use our bodies and spend our time."

Her tips to improve general activity, particularly for those with desk-jobs include:

- Using a standing desk

- Stretching intermittently

- Take calls on a headset so you can stand up or walk around

- Rather than sitting during meetings, find a creative way to keep active (and engaged!) through movement

- Work from home where possible so you have more choice over how you structure your day
- Put in a request for more flexible working hours
- Contribute your ideas on how to make your working environment more dynamic

I realised after my heart attack just how sedentary I had been for most of my working life, and I wanted to do something to change the way I approached my general daily activity.

When my partner used to suggest we take a 5 minute walk to the local shops, I was so conditioned to driving everywhere in a car that I would try to convince her it was too far to walk, or would take too long.

Looking back, I find it shocking that I was so inherently lazy, despite being somebody that would regularly participate in sport.

In January 2020, I decided to try to challenge myself to walk one million steps during the month, as a bit of a shock to my system.

I managed the average 32,258 steps a day to achieve this, and it gave me a great sense of perspective on how little I had moved throughout most of my adult life whilst I had worked in an office.

I calculated, on the days when I have a long drive to my office, and worked at a desk, and then drove home, I averaged about 3,300 steps per day.

Nowadays I make a point of joining my partner Julie for a lunchtime walk for at least an hour, and this along with a morning dog-walk and a few regular "desk-breaks" where I get up and get moving throughout the day, ensures that I average between 15,000 and 20,000 steps per day.

This level of activity has had noticeable effects on my mood, leg strength, blood pressure (8% reduction) and I am sure has dramatically increased the amount of vitamin D I get through sun exposure.

It has also helped increase my metabolism, and will have improved my insulin sensitivity as a result.

Remember N.E.A.T…..and remember being active really adds up to significant health benefits.

HIIT

Nan's Chapter Summary: HIIT is just a term for exercising as hard as you can for a short burst, maybe just for 20 or 30 seconds, and then having a short rest and doing it again a few more times.

There are many benefits from this type of training, like increased endurance and increased strength, as well as being extremely good at improving blood sugar, and emptying big muscles (like the legs) of their built-in stores of glucose.

HIIT can be very stressful on the body, so it is not recommended for everybody. If you want to try HIIT, then speak with your doctor first and always do this kind of training under professional supervision.

Ever heard of High Intensity Interval Training?

HIIT, as it is known, is the performance of a short number of very intense sets of activity, where your heart rate is exercised at roughly 90% of maximum, with short rests between sets.

So, for example…sprinting as fast as possible for 15 seconds, then walking for 45 seconds before doing it again 4 more times would be a 5 set session of HIIT training.

Another example would be cycling on a stationary bicycle, in a tough gear, for 30 seconds as hard as possible, and then taking a 1 minute rest, and repeating this for a number of sets.

When we perform HIIT, we deprive our body of oxygen, and it must adapt to get back to normal. Feeling extremely out of breath after

HIIT is to be expected as our body grabs as much oxygen as it can to return to normal.

Hours after we have completed an HIIT session, our metabolism will still be elevated as our body works to replace nutrients that were lost during the workout.

The positive effects of a HIIT session can still affect our body up to 48 hours after a workout.

One of the things that makes HIIT so valuable is the adaptation our body makes after maximal effort, and the removal of lactic acid build-up, but this can also make it a bit too extreme for many.

Phil Goulding, Senior Personal Trainer at Nuffied Health says;

"HIIT training should be, and is, very hard when performed correctly. This intensity of exercise can be exhilarating, for some and leave you feeling a real sense of accomplishment, but for others it will not be enjoyable".

Often overlooked by those wishing to improve their cardiovascular fitness, HIIT has many additional health benefits that you should be aware of.

Because it requires maximal effort, it strengthens muscles in a similar way to resistance training.

Because it is very intense, and each new set is repeated before your heart rate has returned to normal, it exercises your heart and lungs and increases cardio-vascular endurance.

A study [33] on overweight adults at risk of heart disease concluded;

"HIIT appears to provide similar benefits to MICT (Medium Intensity Continuous Training...like jogging) for improving body composition, VO2 max, but takes less time than MICT in each session."

They went on;

"HIIT is superior to MICT in improving cardio-pulmonary fitness."

Because it takes big muscle groups close to failure, HIIT depletes muscle glycogen stores, and is therefore, very useful at helping to manage blood glucose and improve insulin sensitivity.

Another study[34] concluded;

"HIIT lowered blood glucose and increased exercise capacity, basal activity levels, carbohydrate oxidation and liver and adipose tissue insulin sensitivity."

A 2020 randomised control trial[35] that compared HIIT and standard moderate intensity training to understand the relative benefits for cardiac rehabilitation called ***Comparative Effects of High-Intensity Interval Training vs Moderate-Intensity Continuous***

33
https://journals.plos.org/plosone/article?id=10.1371/journal.pone.0210644

34
https://www.sciencedirect.com/science/article/pii/S2212877815001763

35
https://ideas.repec.org/a/gam/jsusta/v12y2020i10p4134-d359903.html

Training in Phase III of a Tennis-Based Cardiac Rehabilitation Program showed the following interesting results.

"Participants of the HIIT group improved their flexibility in both upper and lower limbs. These results are relevant since a decline in flexibility or agility causes difficulties in performing daily activities."

"In addition, our results showed a significant handgrip strength in favour of the HIIT group. This is quite relevant since grip strength is correlated with mortality and could predict cardiac adverse events in patients with cardiac disorders".

"HIIT appears to provide similar benefits to MICT for improving body composition or cardiorespiratory fitness, which is also in line with previous research".

So the conclusions seem to be, that post-heart attack, where we have a heart that is strong enough to be exercised to high intensity levels (and remember here that a heart attack may be a symptom of blocked arteries and not a weak heart) then there are significantly more benefits to engaging in HIIT activity, or combining it with traditional medium-intensity training such as cycling, walking and jogging, than exercising exclusively at a moderate level.

I would caution though, that if your heart has been significantly damaged by a heart attack, and you have experienced a significant level of necrosis (muscle tissue death), then HIIT activity should be undertaken *only* with supervision, and under advice from your cardiologist.

Working at high intensity should be something that you are sure your heart can cope with, and it is not for the *faint-hearted*, if you excuse the pun.

My particular heart attack, whilst severe in terms of the blockage of the artery, did not cause any significant damage to my heart, and I suffered minimal necrosis, so I feel safe to engage in HIIT activity.

The amount of troponin in your blood after your heart attack will help your cardiologist to understand how much damage your heart has experienced, and this, along with your age, weight, fitness and other factors should be taken into consideration when deciding on the best exercise programme for your recovery.

If you haven't already experienced heart disease and want to massively improve your overall health, I highly recommend HIIT.

Resistance Training

Nan's Chapter Summary: Resistance training includes things like lifting weights, press-ups, using exercise bands. Anything where you are exercising by working against a 'resistance'.

This training method really helps to "empty the bucket" of glucose in your blood, by using up the glucose stored in the muscles, which they then replace by sucking the glucose out of your blood. This helps with blood sugar management.

Resistance training is a term used to describe exercise that involves working against a resistance or load. This covers things like weight training, kettlebell training, using resistance bands, calisthenics (like press-ups, burpees, squat-thrusts) etc.

Resistance training may be something that you have tried before, or it may be completely new to you, but it can play a valuable role in generating great heart health, although maybe not in the way you might think.

Resistance training not only increases your muscle strength, but it also promotes tendon and bone strength, so provides great all-over body benefits.

Additionally, resistance training can increase our muscle mass, and this is particularly good for our hearts.

Firstly, muscles hold their own energy store of glucose. If we increase muscle mass, we increase the amount of glucose that can be stored in the muscles.

This enables our muscles to extract more glucose out of the blood after exercise (when they have been emptied), which as we have discussed, improves insulin sensitivity.

Secondly, an increase in muscle mass automatically increases our body's basal metabolic rate, so we utilise more energy even when we are resting, which again reduces the likelihood of experiencing an excess of energy from food consumed, which will in turn reduce the likelihood of fat storage.

Subcutaneous fat is inflammatory, which is one of the reasons that it is advisable to avoid obesity, and performing regular resistance training is one of the best ways to do this.

If you are worried that, in engaging in resistance training you may start to look like the next Arnold Schwarzenegger, don't!

My first job, after college, was as a weight training instructor, and I often worked with clients who believed that as soon as they lifted a weight they would become "muscle-bound", or "bulky".

It takes many years following a very specific training and dietary regime, with a dedication few can muster, to grow large muscles like a bodybuilder, so there is no need to worry that this will happen.

It is, however, relatively straightforward to start to increase general overall muscle mass, by regularly engaging in resistance training, and your body will benefit from the additional strength, and the improved metabolism that will come with this activity.

There is something that is useful to understand in general when it comes to exercising, and how many calories are "burned" when engaging in resistance training.

It is common for many to believe that going to the gym, or a short run will "burn-off" calories.

There is a temptation to, therefore, "fuel" a workout by eating carbohydrates before training, or reward activity by eating a high-carbohydrate meal after training, and I want to provide a word of caution if this is what you believe to be good practice.

The amount of effort it takes, when engaging in resistance training, to empty muscles of their glycogen stores and then soak up the excess blood glucose from your last meal, is highly likely to be significantly more than most people expend in the gym.

Similarly it is very easy to over-estimate the calories used going for a short run, or session on a bicycle, or a gym session.

Engaging in regular exercise, can often become a justification for "over-indulging" in foods that would otherwise be considered poor choices, and this invariably succeeds in undoing much of the good work that your exercise achieves.

Personal trainers and fitness professionals like to talk about a myriad of ways to manage the intake of carbohydrate, protein, etc around a workout (this is called peri-workout nutrition). They also encourage understanding your calorie deficit/excess each day. This essentially involves their clients weighing and measuring every macronutrient in every meal and trying to consume less calories than they eat every day to lose weight, and the exact amount to maintain weight.

People following these types of regime waste a lot of time living to restrictive recipes, and feeling hungry and weak whilst "accounting" for the amount of protein, carbohydrate and fat in everything they eat.

This is joyless and frustrating, very hard to stick to, and not the best way to nourish your body.

It is also very hard to push through the constant feeling of hunger generated by these eating practices.

There is some validity in the utilisation of the anabolic effects of insulin to assist with muscle development, if you want to become a strength athlete, (or a bodybuilder) but if you don't, this is not a strategy I would advise.

Many such personal trainers believe their clients will not "stick" to a diet without carbohydrates, which is why this type of approach is often suggested. They also have limited understanding of, or thought for, the role of hormones, and the damage caused by excessive insulin.

Having elevated insulin is, however, the single biggest factor in every chronic disease you can think of, and carbohydrates are just sources of glucose, as they are made up from sugars, starches, hydrogen and water. For these reasons this is not an eating method I would recommend.

So do you need carbohydrates to exercise? No you don't.

In the Consumption section, I describe the ketogenic diet.

Following a ketogenic diet does not require weighing and measuring food, counting calories, tracking macronutrients, or anything of the kind.

It just requires a simple understanding of the types of food that you are eating, and trying to make sure that you generally eat foods that provide good nutrient-density, have minimal processing and do not contain sugars and vegetable oils.

It promotes a diet rich in proteins, fats and fruits and vegetables that are high in fibre and have a low glycemic load.

This type of eating style does not elevate insulin and ghrelin, and therefore, does not lead to extreme feelings of hunger.

Studies [36] have shown that overall insulin sensitivity is improved through resistance training, even as little as twice per week.

It has also been shown[37] that resistance training is more effective than aerobic training at improving insulin sensitivity, for the same duration of exercise.

Resistance training also reduces inflammation and helps your body to adapt to utilising ketones as an energy source, which can be easily released from your fat cells, so you have the added benefit of losing body fat, and not needing to calorie-count.

Many people seem to believe that the only type of exercise that is good for the heart is aerobic exercise, but that is a misguided.

Resistance training is a great addition to your activity if you would like to add it.

It is very common knowledge in the sports nutrition and physiology world that a core base of simple, compound resistance training exercises are the bedrock of strength, dynamic power, and overall body health.

These core "Olympic" lifts (as they are known) recruit big muscle groups in your body and they create co-ordination of movement that forms part of good functional patterns for everything we do in life.

These lifts are the deadlift, the squat, the bench press.

Ross Edgley, in his book *The World's Fittest Book* describes his principles how a core base of simple movement patterns that we develop through childhood (running, climbing, jumping and crawling) along with the development of these Olympic-lifts, will create a level of

---

[36]   https://care.diabetesjournals.org/content/21/8/1353.short

[37]   https://www.thieme-connect.com/products/ejournals/abstract/10.1055/s-2007-978828

injury-resilience, force-development and strength that forms the basis for anything else that we choose to do more specifically.

Additionally, because such large muscle groups are activated by these exercises, they "empty the bucket" more efficiently.

This means these are the best exercise to deplete your large muscles of their stored glycogen, meaning any free blood glucose will be sucked-out of the blood to replace it, preventing the need for greater insulin.

My advice would always be to learn these lifts under supervision with a qualified instructor, and learn to add more weight and progress at a sensible rate.

Performing these exercises two to three times a week will improve your strength, improve your co-ordination and help to manage your insulin, so what are you waiting for?

Here are some resistance training tips for optimum insulin sensitivity benefit:

1. Try to engage in at least 3 resistance training sessions each week

2. A good standard protocol is to perform 3 sets of each exercise for between 10 and 15 repetitions

3. Aim to work to "failure" for at least one set of each exercise (more if possible), this means until you literally can't perform one more repetition.

4. Deplete glycogen stores maximally, by engaging in compound exercise that use big muscle groups and multiple body-parts (deadlifts, squats, bench-press, seated rows)

5. Try to maintain good exercise intensity[38] (this is more important than how long you exercise for)

6. Get a personal trainer to help you learn how to use equipment properly and create good technique to ensure you obtain maximum results and avoid injuries

Cardiovascular Exercise

Nan's Chapter Summary: *Cardiovascular exercise just tends to refer to gentle exercise which you can continue comfortably for a while, whilst being slightly out of breath. This is a very safe way to get your heart working during the day without placing it under too much stress.*

Cardiovascular exercise is a term used to describe any activity that gets your heart and lungs working above their normal rate.

There are various different intensities of cardiovascular exercise, or MICT as it is often known.

The different intensity levels are used by athletes to train specifically for either endurance, or maximum oxygen efficiency.

For somebody wishing to strengthen their heart, or just to gain general health benefits, even quite moderate elevation of heart rate can be very effective.

That is why this type of exercise is good to start off rehabilitation after heart disease, or for those that may be older, overweight or infirm.

A good target is to start by walking during the day, for a set period of time, and then gradually increase your walking speed until you are

---

[38]   https://physoc.onlinelibrary.wiley.com/doi/full/10.1113/EP087435

slightly out of breath, and would struggle to hold a conversation, but feel like you are comfortable to continue.

This general level of activity is good for conditioning the heart, but does not create a sense of being overwhelmed.

This type of exercise is by far the most common form of rehabilitation exercise after a heart attack.

Whilst you may decide to take-up cycling or jogging, I generally like to think of this type of exercise as an extension of NEAT. Even though many may class it as specific exercise, to me it is an extension of having an active lifestyle, which is extremely beneficial.

Sun

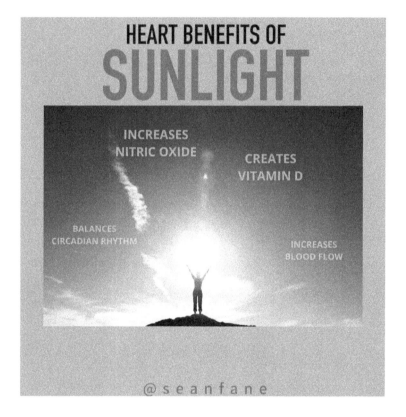

The **S** in C.R.A.S.H. is Sun.

One of the first things we learn about the earth in school is how the planet and its various organisms need water and the sun for survival.

In fact the earth would not have developed at all without its proximity to the sun.

It is the earth's relationship to the sun, and the amount of light it receives, that is responsible for the seasons and biodiversity. The amount of sun a region receives depends on the tilt of the earth's axis, and it is

316

easy to see what life is able to be sustained at the areas that receive the least quantities.

How long do you think any of us would last if we were dropped-off naked at the North or South Pole?

Not long!

When we later study plants in biology classes, for example, we are taught that for photosynthesis to take place, plants need 3 things; to take in carbon dioxide (from the air), water (from the ground) and light (usually from the sun, but of course now we can make artificial light for plants to grow day and night).

I was taught that humans have 5 basic needs for survival; air, water, nutrients (food), sleep and shelter (if you presume that with all of the other elements we may die from extremes of weather).

The omission from this list, and it's a big one, is sunlight.

When you think about a human's basic nutritional requirements, you begin to realise that all of the foods from which we derive nutrition (animals and plants) to some extent rely on the sun.

Eat beef?

A cow can't live without grass, which requires the sun for photosynthesis.

Eat plants?

…..you get the picture.

The Sun warms our seas, stirs our atmosphere, generates our weather patterns, and gives energy to the plants that provide the food and oxygen for life on Earth.

But do humans need sunlight more directly than as a function of creating the planet in which we live and providing the basis for all of the food we eat?

Do we actually need direct sunlight ourselves to survive?

It turn's out, sunlight is a lot like food in that it facilitates chemical processes, supports hormones, and enables us to express our genes.

Being out in the open air is a necessity. We weren't designed to spend our lives wrapped-up in clothes.

There is so much confusion and mis-information about sun exposure that many people only feel safe, relaxed and comfortable by covering-up when going outside.

Whether we are conforming to a social need to be dressed "formally" or Victorian values of decency, we wear long sleeves and trousers and cover large parts of our bodies most of the time.

In some cultures, there is a religious and cultural imperative to cover almost the entire body (especially for women).

In others, there is a cultural norm that considers darker skin as less attractive, so sun exposure is avoided in order to keep a complexion as "fair" as possible. An 2014 marketing study on Indian girls[39] noted that almost 90% of Indian girls cite skin lightening as a "high need".

Then there is of course, the more recent phenomenon of almost paranoia relating to the potential for skin cancer from excessive sun exposure, and for many people the desire to delay the potential for any ageing effect from sun exposure on their faces.

Whatever the reason, sun exposure has never been so unpopular.

---

[39] https://theconversation.com/bleached-girls-india-and-its-love-for-light-skin-80655

Our bodies thrive in natural sunlight, and even a small amount every day stimulates collagen production, which is clearly very good for the skin.

We have, over time, eroded some of our bodies defences against many threats (through poor dietary choices and modern agriculture) and sun exposure seems to be one of them.

Stephanie Seneff - is a senior research scientist at the Computer Science and Artificial Intelligence Laboratory (CSAIL) of the Massachusetts Institute of Technology (MIT).

In 2013, Seneff co-authored a paper that associated the herbicide glyphosate with a wide variety of diseases such as cancer and disorders such as autism.

Glyphosate also damages some of the healthy gut bacteria that enable us produce more of the compounds that protect us from sun damage.

Contrary to common understanding there is also actually a strong correlation between sunscreen use and risks from melanoma.

The Journal of the American Academy of Dermatology has stated.

"Sunscreen is a multibillion-dollar industry, and its efficacy in the prevention of skin cancer is often taken as fact. Despite this, there are only four prospective studies that examine sunscreen's role in preventing skin cancer, and none of these studies examine the efficacy of sunscreen in preventing skin cancer in otherwise healthy individuals."

"Melanoma, is a complex disease: Genetics, patterns of exposure (regular sun exposure may be less harmful than intermittent, high-intensity sunlight, for example), and other still-unknown factors contribute to the risk. This may partly explain why melanoma rates in the U.S. have tripled since the 1970s, even as the use of sunscreen has increased."

Melanin, which is our bodies in-built protection from the harmful effects of sunlight, is made out of cross-linked polyphenols, so a diet rich in these powerful anti-oxidants helps you build a strong system to harness the suns health-boosting effects without exposing yourself to any harmful rays.

And where skin cancer is concerned, a report on sunscreens from Environmental Working Group (EWG), a non-profit consumer watchdog, stated;

"Insufficient evidence exists to prove that sunscreen actually helps prevent skin cancer."

Great! So what are we using it for.

Additionally, one of the suspected risk factors in skin cancer (as well as other types of cancer and numerous other health problems) is vitamin D deficiency, caused by too *little* sun exposure!

As you can imagine, this is a natural process. We did, after all, thrive and evolve on a planet with the same sun that we have now for thousands of years before sunscreen and Victorian values arrived.

Getting back to nature and getting outside, are part of becoming a more resilient, happy and healthy human..

Want to feel great and protect your heart?

Get Naked!

Let's consider what chemical processes actually occur when sunlight is absorbed by our skin….it's quite interesting.

The two main benefits of sunlight can be categorised as vitamin D production and nitric oxide (NO) production.

Let's start with vitamin D.

Vitamin D

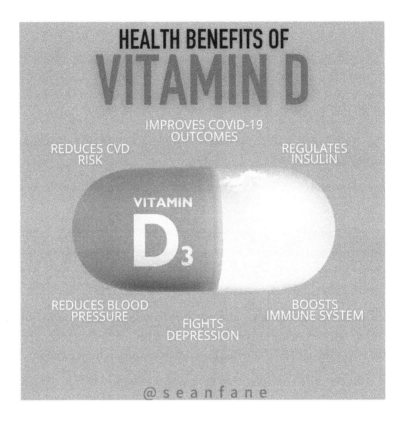

Nan's Chapter Summary: Vitamin D can be obtained from food, but the majority we obtain from sun exposure.

If we limit our exposure to direct sunlight, by applying sun-cream, wearing clothes or just staying indoors, we reduce the amount of vitamin D we obtain.

Vitamin D is vital for immune health and strong bones, but also for producing a lot of the hormones that are responsible for us thriving.

Low vitamin D is associated with heart disease, and increased suscep-tibility to illnesses.

Vitamin D is sometimes called the "sunshine vitamin" because it's produced in our skin in response to sunlight exposure. It's a fat-soluble vitamin in a family of compounds that includes vitamins D-1, D-2, and D-3.

It isn't technically a vitamin, it is a pre-hormone, used to help produce other hormones.

Our bodies produce vitamin D naturally when our skin is exposed to sunlight.

We can also obtain it through certain foods, such as eggs, salmon, sardines, red meat, liver, mushrooms and from supplements to ensure adequate levels of the vitamin in your blood, but the majority is obtained through sun exposure.

Once sunlight enters the body from the skin, or we obtain vitamin D through our diet, it is converted by the liver into something called 25(OH) Vitamin D, which can then be fully utilised by your cells.

Every cell in our body has a vitamin D receptor.

Vitamin D regulates anti-body activity and immune function, so it is an important part of keeping well and defending us from bacteria, infections and viruses.

It also regulates the absorption of calcium and phosphorus, without which our bones would crumble.

This is why obtaining a sufficient amount of vitamin D is important for normal growth and development of bones and teeth, as well as improved resistance against certain diseases.

Macrophages, little organisms that "gobble-up" bacteria and viruses, are activated with vitamin D.

In 2006 it was discovered that macrophages, signal cells to produce a protein called cathelicidin, which specifically kills infectious agents like Tuberculosis and Coronavirus.

Some of vitamin D's protective super-powers were known as long ago as 1849, when cod liver oil was used to help beat Tuberculosis by virtue of its vitamin D content.

Vitamin D helps adaptive immunity protection for COVID-19, but also helps prevent contracting it in the first place through interaction with the angiotensin receptors, which is how COVID-19 can access the body.

A study on 160,000 people has shown…..being vitamin D sufficient (above 60 ng/ml v 20 ng/ml) reduces COVID-19 risk by 54% [40].

It also resists cancer cells.

If you google vitamin D and cancer, you will be bombarded by studies and tests that show the effects of improving cancer treatment with vitamin D.

And lastly, vitamin D reduces insulin resistance, and if you read the whole of this book (as I hope you will) you will understand how important for heart health this is.

Vitamin D is cumulative, but if your body doesn't get enough in the summer, (particularly if you live in the northern hemisphere and/or you have skin with darker pigment which absorbs less UVB rays from the sun) you will have depleted levels through the darker winter months, and be more susceptible to infections and viruses.

---

[40] https://www.bumc.bu.edu/busm/2020/09/25/adequate-levels-of-vitamin-d-reduces-complications-death-among-covid-19-patients/

This is why it is very important to top-up vitamin D in the summer as much as possible, to see you through the winter...... or alternatively supplement throughout the winter, when your levels would otherwise drop.

It is no coincidence that in the winter, when blood levels of vitamin D are at their lowest, respiratory tract infections are at their highest.

There is apparently no downside to additional vitamin D.

Too much, can be a problem, but is difficult to achieve. The main consequence of vitamin D toxicity is a buildup of calcium in your blood (hypercalcemia). It is estimated that to do this one would need to supplement with 60,000 iu per day for many months, so would be a self-inflicted issue.

A growing number of studies point to vitamin D deficiency as a risk factor for heart attacks, heart failure, peripheral arterial disease, strokes, and the conditions associated with cardiovascular disease, such as high blood pressure and diabetes.

The definition of vitamin D deficiency in the UK is under 10 ng/ml in the blood, but this is very, very low.

Good bone health requires 40 ng/ml as a bare minimum, and there is good evidence to support 40-60 ng/ml being a reasonable target level. As you will learn, there are some that think this is still a very low-level though.

To get your vitamin D levels topped-up through diet is quite tough, and you may need to supplement at high doses initially to nudge your blood levels up to close to 60 ng/ml.

Dr Judson Somerville wrote a book on his, and his patients, life-changing impacts from high-dose vitamin D supplementation, called **The Optimal Dose**.

He suggests a protocol to increase circulating vitamin D to good levels, of 20,000 iu per day for six weeks and then reduction to 10,000 iu until blood levels reach 50-60 ng/ml.

He also, however, explains that optimal benefits from vitamin D come from a circulating blood level of between 100-140 ng/ml, and this he suggests is achieved by supplementing with 30,000 iu per day and then testing your levels and reducing to a maintenance dose once you are in this range.

Ignore the RDA for vitamin D. It was set at the lowest dose of vitamin D that will prevent rickets....not a level that will provide good health.

Somerville suggests in his book that low circulating vitamin D can predicate weight gain.

This seems to take effect by signalling to the body that it is "going into winter", encouraging fat stores to accumulate to accommodate less food and the cold weather.

He suggests that those with optimum circulating vitamin D levels have incredibly robust immune function, feel less cravings and hunger, find it easier to lose weight, improve their sleep dramatically and create hormonal balance that supports many other positive physiological outcomes.

I don't know about you, but I think that this makes direct sunlight pretty much an essential for life. Certainly a life without a lot of issues.

Tips to ensure you have optimum vitamin D levels:

1. *Eat your vitamin D* - Make eggs, oily fish and mushrooms a key component of your diet.

2. *Get out in the sun* - Spend at least 20 minutes a day with your skin exposed to the sun, without sunscreen.

3. ***Supplement (especially in winter)*** - Vitamin D is a cheap supplement, so make sure you get at least 4,000 iu a day as a supplement.

4. ***Take a bigger dose!*** - Increase your vitamin D intake to up 30,000 iu per day for a few days if you have a cold or flu (or if you want to get to Dr Judson Somerville's recommended levels). Additional supplementation with vitamin D has been shown to have al almost antibiotic-like effect when you are feeling very run-down.

The other benefit from sunlight I mentioned was nitric oxide.

Don't worry…this is a quick one.

Nitric Oxide

Nitric oxide is produced by nearly every type of cell in the human body and is one of the most important molecules for blood vessel health.

It is a vasodilator, meaning it relaxes the inner muscles of our blood vessels, causing them to widen.

In this way, nitric oxide increases blood flow and lowers blood pressure, which is extremely positive for our cardiovascular system.

UVA rays from the sun release nitric oxide from the skin, and have been shown to significantly improve cardiovascular health.

A 2014 paper [41] highlighting the role of nitric oxide concluded;

---

[41]
https://www.sciencedirect.com/science/article/pii/S0022202X153
68974

"The report describes a hitherto unrecognised role for this compound (nitric oxide) in reducing the risk factors for cardiovascular disease."

Improved blood flow, and oxygen delivery, are reasons why nitric oxide is considered useful for performance athletes, and is why some athletes opt to drink beetroot juice before an endurance event. Beetroot juice is high in nitrates, and our body converts nitrates into nitric oxide.

Due to its effects in increasing nitric oxide and improving blood flow, the chaps reading this may be interested to know that beetroot juice is often recommended for those that suffer with erectile dysfunction.

Good blood flow works for more than one organ in the body.

Lastly on the sun.....getting-out in the sun makes us feel good.

It is a mood enhancer.

Mood Enhancer

It makes us feel relaxed and happy when we have the warm sun radiating on our back.

This is a chemical response, and not just imagined.

Exposure to sunlight is thought to increase the brain's release of a hormone called serotonin. Serotonin is associated with boosting mood and helping us feel calm and focused.

Many people refer to seasonal affective disorder (SAD), which is when one feels low, down or depressed in the winter months. There is clinical evidence of the sun's positive impact on mental health to support the validity of SAD when we are deprived of sunlight.

In a 2009 article entitled *Effect of sunlight exposure on cognitive function among depressed and non-depressed participants*[42] it was found that there was;

"An association between decreased exposure to sunlight and increased probability of cognitive impairment using a novel data source."

Those suffering anxiety and depression are at higher risk of heart disease, due to the negative impact these conditions have on hormonal balance, so improving these mental health aspects through sunlight exposure has a significant impact on our heart health.

The take-home message for this section is to ditch the sun-cream, and get some sun. Just don't allow yourself to burn.

At least 20 minutes of direct sunlight on your skin each day is recommended to help maintain vitamin D levels, and this is significantly less than most of us get.

Whether we are darker skinned people living in the Northern hemisphere, or lighter skinned people protecting ourselves from burns or worrying about skin cancer, we spend most of our lives covered-up by clothes or slathered in creams with an SPF of 8 or more, impairing our own ability to benefit from the greatest source of life and vitality there is.

I can't think of many things more counter-productive for our health.

Embrace the sun, it is your heart's friend.

---

[42] https://link.springer.com/article/10.1186/1476-069X-8-34

HORMONES

The *H* in C.R.A.S.H. is Hormones.

I will only talk about two hormones, but as master hormones that recruit many others to assist in their work, managing these two effectively, will also enable many others to remain balanced within your body.

Insulin

Nan's Chapter Summary: *Reducing insulin by eating a diet low in sugar and carbohydrates, exercising regularly, and keeping active is extremely important to create a hormone balance which supports good heart health.*

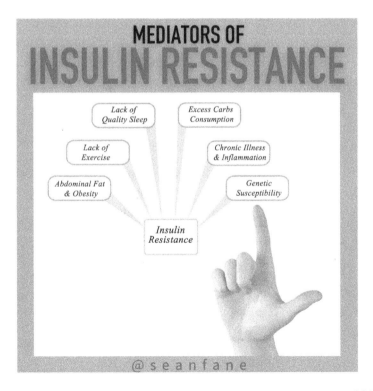

I have written a lot about insulin resistance and its importance as the catalyst of many chronic health conditions.

It is vitally important for anabolic activity (muscle growth. And development) and for clearing glucose from your bloodstream, before it can wreak too much havoc.

It is also the driver for insulin resistance, through the lifestyle habit we have created of eating foods with a high glycemic load, and eating too frequently.

One of the cornerstones of the **H** in the CRASH system is to minimise the secretion of insulin.

There are a number of ways to achieve this, reduce circulating insulin and improve insulin sensitivity.

The first is to eat a ketogenic diet.

This is a diet that consists of no more than 20g of carbohydrates a day, and where foods with a low glycemic load are prioritised over their nutrient poor, high-glycemic counterparts.

This is a diet which will limit hunger, reduce inflammation, improve insulin sensitivity and create a stable environment from which our body can repair any damage to our cardiovascular system.

I won't add anything further, except remind you that insulin is the architect of our metabolic pain, and the gang leader of a number of other hormones, that it recruits in order to help with its dirty work.

Cortisol

Nan's Chapter Summary: *Reducing cortisol by relaxing, meditating, socialising with friends and family and practicing gratitude is extremely important to create a hormone balance to support your heart health.*

One of the other hormonal gang leaders is cortisol.

Cortisol is produced mainly in the adrenal gland, but also in other tissues in lower quantities.

It is released in response to stress and low blood-glucose concentrations.

It functions to increase blood (sugar through gluconeogenesis), to suppress the immune system, and to aid in the metabolism of fat, protein, and carbohydrates.

It works along with norepinephrine (noradrenaline) as part of what is referred to as the "fight or flight" response, which is the sympathetic nervous systems response to perceived threat or danger.

Whether triggered by a hungry lion heading towards us, or a pending deadline, our body's response to stress can be both helpful and harmful.

The stress response gives us the strength and speed to ward off, or flee, from an impending threat (increasing blood sugar, increasing blood pressure, increasing senses, increasing heart rate, reducing immune function and digestion, etc). This is great for a short-term escape from danger.

When it occurs frequently, however, stress can put us at risk for obesity, heart disease, cancer, and a variety of other illnesses.

In a 2020 article on the Physiology of the Stress Response[43], the authors described how chronically elevated cortisol affects immune function;

"If the stressful event persists for extended periods of time, the body will adapt to cope with the higher level of stress. The body will continue to secrete stress hormones

---

43   https://www.ncbi.nlm.nih.gov/books/NBK541120/

which keep the body's physical response to stress elevated. This induces the resistance stage and includes symptoms of poor concentration, irritability, and frustration. If the stressful event continues to persist further, the body will enter the exhaustion stage. Symptoms of this stage include burnout, fatigue, depression, anxiety, and reduced stress tolerance. As the stressful event persists, the body's immune system will continue to weaken. This is due to the suppressive effects of stress hormone on cells of the immune system."

As mentioned in the section on recuperation, minimising stressors and anxiety is key to reducing cortisol, which in turn will limit circulating blood glucose and help improve insulin sensitivity.

Techniques that limit your production of cortisol are another hormonal cornerstone of recovery, and prevention of heart disease, and are outlined in the Recuperation section.

HABIT FORMING - HOW TO STICK TO ANYTHING

One of the challenges I always encounter when I have read a book containing good ideas for personal development, is that I remember one or two practical things I could incorporate into my life, but I forget the rest.

After a period of trying to incorporate the few habits I remember, I usually find it difficult to keep momentum in practicing them, until eventually I wake up one morning realising that I have gotten out of the habit altogether.

I knew that after my heart attack I was going to need to demonstrate far more "will-power" than usual, and really make some permanent changes to my lifestyle, so I started to learn a few life-hacks on how to remember things better, and how to create habits I could stick to.

The image below is my version of the bicycle made famous by Mattias Ribbing, who is sometimes referred to as Grand Master of Memory.

USE YOUR HEAD, HEAL YOUR HEART
Ribbings Bike

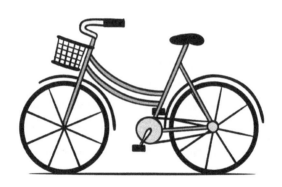

Ribbing created a great technique, to help people remember 10 items really easily.

He asks us to picture a bicycle, maybe our current bike — whatever we can visualise in detail.

Next he asks us to enlarge it in our mind, and picture it right in front of us.

If you are doing this now, think of maybe up to 10 things you need to remember, things like the elements of C.R.A.S.H. for example;

For Consumption: Foods to eat (picture butter & meat for example) supplements to take (picture a supplement pill), pollutants (picture a factory)

For Recuperation: Yoga (a yogi in a pose), somebody meditating, sleep (a pillow)

For Activity: NEAT (a hiker), Resistance training (dumbbell)

For Sun: The Sun

For Hormones: Exercise (dumbbell), foods to avoid (bread, sugar), Insulin (syringe), connection (people together)

USE YOUR HEAD, HEAL YOUR HEART
C.R.A.S.H.

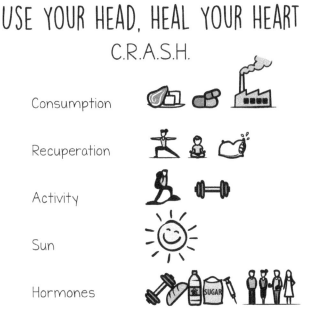

Consumption

Recuperation

Activity

Sun

Hormones

Now try to imagine these elements in a cartoonish, outlandish or funny style placed on one of 10 different locations on Ribbings Bike from left to right;

1. Maybe starting with the basket at the front, full of healthy food

2. Then the front spokes might be a dumbbell

3. The frame has a yogi in a pose

4. The pedal is a pillow

5. There is a chap meditating on the pillow

6. The saddle is a supplement

7. A hiker is standing on top of the supplements

8. The rear mudguard has your friends on it

9. Falling off the back of the bike are all the toxins you want to remove from your life, bread, sugar, insulin syringe

10. The Sun is smiling down on you from behind the bike

Here is an example of how this might look.

USE YOUR HEAD, HEAL YOUR HEART
Ribbings Bike

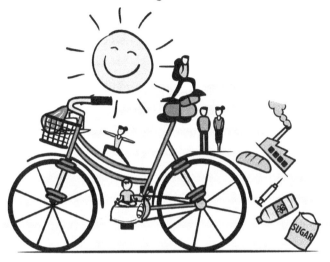

The more fun, and comical, you make the image in your head of the items on your bike, the more likely you are to be able to recall them when you think of the bike.

This incredibly simple little memory tool has helped me to keep in mind the various elements of my lifestyle that I wanted to focus on.

The next challenge was, how to "stick" to them, which is a little more challenging.

We all have a little morning routine.

Yours may be slightly different to mine, but there are a few things that most people will do every day when they wake up.

We may take a shower, brush our teeth, have a shave, get dressed and then head to the kitchen for breakfast.

When was the last time you heard somebody forget to have a shower?....or complain that shampoo was really expensive?....or get frustrated at the time it takes to brush their teeth?

This funny little routine, that we all develop as children, and continue through our lives, is never considered too much trouble, and we take for granted the massive cumulative effect that it has.

Our teeth last significantly longer (especially with the diets we have these days) than they otherwise would, we have made body odour virtually extinct (which I am sure we all agree is a good thing), we look and feel better as a consequence of these daily tasks, and we pretty much never forget to do them.

Think for a minute how you would look and feel if for a month you didn't; shower, use deodorant, brush your teeth, shampoo your hair or choose new clothes to wear each day.

A pretty grim thought, I am sure you agree!

What about if you didn't do this for a whole year?

Heaven forbid!

What about 10 years!!?

It is hard to imagine anything other than a complete decline in your appearance, smell, personal hygiene and mental as well as physical health.

The psychology of how we form the habits that become intrinsic parts of our lives is very interesting.

If we could create heart-health habits as well practiced as our morning routine, that didn't seem intrusive, where we never gave a second thought to the time, money or effort they took to complete (because they were just part of our lives) then we would never really have to worry about heart disease too much.

In his great book ***Atomic Habits*** James Clear explains the principles of forming good habits, and outlines what we can do to ensure that the little life-hacks that we want to add into our lives really stick.

His motto is *"Tiny changes, remarkable results!"*

You might look through the C.R.A.S.H. programme and see that there are a number of things that you might want to incorporate into your life, but which could be difficult to do consistently, or stick-to over time.

Clear has a few great tips on how to create habits and stick to them, and I have found these really useful when trying to implement things like;

- Taking supplements

- Meditating

- Exercising

- Drinking enough water

- Remembering to eat healthy food

- Getting enough good-quality sleep

So what are the key elements to creating habits and sticking with them?

1. ***Make it obvious*** - Clear suggests that if you want to remember to do something, then makes it really obvious. An example would be to leave your yoga mat in front of the sink in the bathroom. Then every morning when you go to brush your teeth, you will see the yoga mat and be reminded to get some practice in before getting ready for your day. If you want to perform resistance training in the evening, leave your gym kit by

the front door in the morning, so that they are the first thing you see when you come home after work.

2. **Make it attractive** - If you want to run for exercise every day, then go and buy yourself some really nice running shoes and a track suit that you love wearing. Let your friends know that you want to go running, and see if any want to join you. The more fun and attractive you make the experience the more you will want to participate in it.

3. **Make it easy** - Just like making something obvious, making it easy really helps. If I want to use weights for resistance training after work each day, but the nearest gym is a 20 minute drive in the wrong direction from my journey from the office back home, then the chances of me sticking to a gym routine are pretty slim. If I join a gym close to my office, or have a set of weights at home, then I am more likely to exercise as it will be much more convenient.

4. **Make it satisfying** - Give yourself a reward for sticking to your new habit each day. If, for example, you decide to only allow yourself a coffee after you have completed one of your new habits, then it will not only help to remind you to perform the habit, but will also start to associate the habit with a morning cup of coffee, which will make the habit more enjoyable.

5. **Habit Stacking** - This is a great tip. Stack more than one habit together…this way they become a little set of routines you remember to perform one after the other, and they are more likely to be achieved. A great example is, if you want to listen to a podcast or audio book for an hour every day, and you also want to increase your step-count and general activity, why not go for a 45 minute walk every day while listening to the podcast! That is a 2-for-1 habit stack!

These are just a few tips on how to create new habits and stick to them, but I highly recommend James' book if you want to learn more about forming new heart healthy habits.

WHAT YOU MUST DO IF YOU ARE LUCKY ENOUGH TO SURVIVE A HEART ATTACK

WHEN YOU LEAVE HOSPITAL

If you have experienced a heart attack, then firstly let me say that I am sorry that you have been through such an ordeal.

When you leave hospital you may, understandably, feel vulnerable and scared.

You may also feel confused about what the future holds for you, and you will certainly have been prescribed a package of drugs to take, some temporarily, but some for the rest of your life.

You will also be given some advice on lifestyle interventions you can take, some of this advice is good and some I have found is poor.

If you are based in the UK it is likely that you will be given a lifestyle protocol that will incorporate minimising cholesterol in your diet, performing light exercise daily, and attending a cardiac rehabilitation programme at an out-patient hospital.

Frustratingly, I found that I was placed in a class of elderly men and women. Our, exercise routine was extremely pedestrian, and consisted of stepping from side-to-side for 2 minutes, then resting, then lifting 2 pound dumbbells for 20 seconds, then resting, along with a couple of other exercises of a similar level.

I would encourage you not to be too frustrated with this approach if you are younger and more mobile than the average level of the class you are in.

A slow start is certainly to be recommended, even if you are feeling pretty normal, but when you and your cardiologist agree that your heart is coping well with going up and down through exercise ranges, you should start to tailor your programme specifically to you.

You may experience hyper-vigilance. This is the annoying experience where you pay super-attention to every feeling you have in your chest, panicking that you might have another heart attack. This is very upsetting and stressful. I experienced this periodically throughout the first year after my heart attack!

Of those that experience a heart attack, roughly 20% will go on to have another heart attack within 5 years of their first.

It is possible for issues to arise with blood clotting from stents, so dual anti-platelet therapy (DAPT) is provided after stenting. However, if the DAPT is continued for more than 30 months there can be increased risk of internal bleeding. The path post-heart attack is not smooth.

I do not say this to scare you. I hope that you will be able to find a good balance between being aware of what is happening within your body, whilst not feeling too anxious. You have a second chance at life, so don't waste it panicking.

You should let your partner, friends and loved-ones know if you feel you have any further symptoms, so you can be assessed, and if necessary, treated quickly.

It may be comforting to know that with the right lifestyle interventions and a good awareness of how to deal with any potential challenges, you can live a very full, long and productive life after a heart attack.

Whilst you may feel re-assured by following medical advice and taking drugs that have been prescribed, some of the medications have little or no efficacy, and some may increase your risk of heart disease, and also result in a long list of side effects.

I do not want to suggest to you that you should entirely reject your medical advice.

Instead, I would like you to feel well-informed and able to question the things you are told by your medical practitioners, so that you can make the best decisions for your future.

Whilst I was learning about the efficacy of statins, for example, I did still take them.

In fact, I carried-on taking them for about 2 months after I discovered their lack of efficacy.

I guess I was hedging-my-bets. I hadn't been on them for long enough for side effects to show, and I was afraid of the consequences for my health of going against doctors advice.

Once I had read sufficiently, examined the evidence thoroughly, and the conclusions were very clear, I had the confidence to stop taking statins.

Despite the fact that I fall into the one category of patient where there is a small benefit for statins (by reducing inflammation), I concluded that I can reduce my inflammatory much better through other lifestyle changes, and I don't want to open myself up to any of the side effects of statins.

Here is a list of the medications I was prescribed when leaving hospital, and why they were administered. You may be prescribed similar:

- To lower cholesterol: **Atorvastatin** (despite the fact that this does not decrease CVD risk)

- To lower blood pressure: **Ramipril** (despite the fact that my blood pressure was in the normal range)

- To prevent blood clotting: **Clopidogrel** (anti platelet used in conjunction with Aspirin in what is called DAPT - dual anti platelet therapy. This is a common prescription after a stent is fitted to prevent the new stent from creating blood clots which can be dangerous. Advice is to continue DAPT for at least 12 months.)

- To "thin" the blood: **Aspirin** (For people who have already had a heart attack or stroke, taking aspirin daily for two years prevented 1 in 50 from having a further cardiovascular problem)

- To manage some of the stomach issues from the above medications: **Ranitidine**

These are the NHS listed side effects for the drugs I was prescribed:

Atorvastatin: **Statin**

Feeling sick (nausea) or indigestion, headaches, aches and pains in your back and joints, nosebleeds, sore throat, cold-like symptoms, such as a runny nose, blocked nose or sneezing, constipation or wind, diarrhoea, muscle pain, tenderness, weakness or cramps **(signs of muscle breakdown and kidney damage)**, yellow skin or the whites of your eyes turn yellow, or if you have pale faeces and dark urine **(sign of liver problems)**, a skin rash with pink-red blotches, especially on the palms of the hands or soles of the feet, severe stomach pain (this can be a sign of pancreas problems), a cough, feeling short of breath, and weight loss **(sign of lung disease)**, a serious allergic reaction (anaphylactic shock).

The NHS website misses out the following known issues: The promotion of **type 2 diabetes**, development of **cancer**, development of neurodegenerative diseases, **Alzheimer's**, **dementia**, **impotence** in men, **reduced sex-drive** in women, **depression**, exacerbation of symptoms of asthma, etc. For further reading on the studies highlighting these issues relative to statins refer to Statins Toxic Side Effects by David Evans.

Ramipril: **ACE Inhibitor**

Dry, tickly cough that does not go away, feeling dizzy or light-headed, headaches, diarrhoea, vomiting, a mild skin rash, blurred vision, yellow skin or the whites of your eyes turn yellow (a sign of liver problems), paleness, tiredness, faint or dizzy, bleeding (like bleeding from the gums and bruising more easily), sore throat, high temperature, greater susceptibility to infections (signs of a blood or bone marrow disorder), **faster heart rate, chest pain and tightness in your chest (signs of heart problems)**, shortness of breath and wheezing (signs of lung problems), severe stomach pain (sign of an inflamed pancreas), swollen ankles, blood in urine or inability to urinate – these can be (signs of kidney problems), **weak arms and legs or problems speaking (signs of a stroke)**.

Clopidogrel: *Antiplatelet*

Bleeding more easily than normal - nosebleeds, bruising more easily or bleeding that takes longer to stop, diarrhoea, stomach pain, indigestion or heartburn.

Aspirin: *Blood Thinner*

Indigestion, nosebleeds, red, blistered and peeling skin, coughing up blood or blood in your urine, faeces or vomit, yellow skin or the whites of your eyes turn yellow (sign of liver problems), painful joints in the hands and feet (sign of high levels of uric acid in the blood), swollen hands or feet (sign of water retention)

Ranitidine: *Histamine Antagonist*

Stomach pains, constipation, feeling sick, stomach pain that seems to be getting worse (sign of an inflamed liver or pancreas), back pain, fever, pain when peeing or blood in your pee (signs of kidney problems), rash, swollen joints or kidney problems (signs that your small blood vessels are swollen), slow or irregular heartbeat (signs of heart problems).

Ranitidine is no longer available through the NHS.

As of writing this, the NHS website posts the following statement for Ranitidine:

Ranitidine is not currently available in the UK. There is an ongoing investigation into whether some ingredients can increase the risk of cancer. All supplies have been stopped until the medicine is shown to be safe.

Is it too much to ask that medicine is not prescribed at all until it is shown to be safe!?

If you are unsure about whether a medication you have been prescribed is safe or effective, there are a number of places where you can research the efficacy and side effects.

Use all of the resources at your disposal to ensure you can make the right choice.

www.askapatient.com is an example of a website where you can enter a medication, and it will provide results of feedback from patients taking that medication. Patients often explain any side effects they have experienced as well as whether the medication seemed to help with their symptoms.

YOUR MENTAL HEALTH

Nan's Chapter Summary: Please try not to be too anxious after recovering from your heart attack.

You will have been through a frightening ordeal, but worrying about heart disease is not likely to help you to recover well.

As hard as it may seem, try to feel gratitude and excitement every day, and think of this as a second chance at life.

Be kind to yourself, and treat yourself the way you would one of your friends if they suffered in the same way.

Take positive little steps each day towards a good recovery.

One of the aspects of life after a heart attack that doesn't seem to receive much consideration, is the effect it can have on one's mental health.

This seems very strange to me, as it has long been understood that stress, loneliness, anxiety and depression are significant risk factors for developing heart disease in the first place.

Once released from hospital after a heart-attack (I refer to the UK as this is the only experience I have to go on) one is advised to:

- Take more exercise (but not over-exert oneself)

- Eat less fat and cholesterol (terrible advice)

- Quit smoking (if applicable)

- Don't expose yourself to extremes of temperature

- Reduce stress (although if the stress comes from an intrinsic part of your pre heart attack life, such as your job, your relationship or money worries, then that is easier said than done).

For many, this advice leads one on a path of life adjustment and improved health practices.

Some of my rehabilitation cohort had goals such as; increase their step-count to aim for 10,000 steps a day, lose the 2/3/4 stone they have been carrying around for a while, and clean-up their poor eating practices (although in this, the advice sometimes leads them down a counter-productive path).

The big elephant-in-the-room that seems to go completely un-noticed, however, is the thing common to all heart-attack survivors?

What do all heart-attack survivors have in common?

They all have the knowledge, and accompanying stress of knowing that they nearly died from cardio-vascular disease, and there is a very strong likelihood that they will experience another event. This is enough to make anybody anxious and depressed.

Heart disease isn't something that occurs overnight.

Everybody that experiences heart disease has had an internal environment that has been progressively compromised over a long period of time to result in their myocardial infarction or stroke.

Some of that may be genetic, some may be environmental and some may be their poor lifestyle practices, but all survivors will be left with a puzzle to solve. Which elements of their lifestyle and genetics created their heart disease and which are, therefore, priorities to redress in the hope that this may delay (or prevent) a recurrence.

This leads to big challenges in terms of life adjustment. Changing things that have become normal behaviours for decades is really, really hard.....even if the consequences of doing nothing are terminal.

I know this first-hand, as I still find myself mindlessly ordering fish and chips cooked in a deep fat fryer, despite knowing the inflammatory burden that vegetable oil will put on my cardiovascular system.

If a 65 year old male that lives alone and has a poor social life, smokes 60 cigarettes and drinks 3 litres of Coca Cola a day and is 6 stone overweight, survives a heart attack, then there are a number of very obvious changes that can be made to improve his chances of another event.

The fact that he has gone through years of this type of physical self-abuse, and has such obvious risk-factors means that losing weight, cessation of smoking and removing sugar will have a massive impact on his condition. This won't be easy, especially as the habits that he has developed may have been ingrained over many years.

How much harder would it be then, for the survivor of a heart attack that doesn't smoke, has a vibrant social-life and lives with a loving partner, isn't overweight, eats well, exercises regularly and is relatively young?

Not only are there lifestyle/environmental changes that must be made for these people, but they probably don't know what those might be. They may also need to take more extreme measures than those with more obvious risk-factors, to mitigate future heart-health issues.

For example....if a genetic pre-disposition for clotting, or a genetically high LP(a) level is present in a survivor, that person knows that they 'can't afford' to adopt what most would consider a generally "healthy" lifestyle. They may need to be more careful.

Simple lifestyle interventions may not be enough. They may not even be aware of the habits in their previous lifestyle which might have prevented their heart-disease from developing.

They may need to adopt a very strict dietary regime (such as a ketogenic diet), give-up a job they love (if the accompanying stress might have been a factor in their disease) and have many subsequent potential lifestyle changes as a result of this (such as down-sizing their home and other financial sacrifices).

These are big decisions.

They may need to take very specific supplements, and regularly measure their risk factors with blood tests.

With all of these challenges to address, they may have no real understanding of whether it will make any difference, because the UK medical system seems to have no answer to the reasonable question *"what was it that caused my heart-attack?" ......other than* "It must be genetic. We don't know the cause! You don't have any risk factors."

One in five heart-attack survivors will have another one within 5 years of the first.

Imagine how that would affect your mental health if it was you that had survived a heart attack.

The thought that you nearly died, you were saved this time, but you are likely to have the experience repeated again.

Now imagine the medical professionals treating you have no idea what caused it, and have no interest in going through an exploratory process to find out either.

The protocol in the UK in these instances is to prescribe the highest dose of statins available (80mg Atorvastatin for me) even though there is no evidence that they prevent heart-attacks and they actually increase all-cause mortality (death), as well as potentially delivering a slew of horrible side-effects including Alzheimer's, dementia, muscle pain, joint-pain, diabetes and erectile dysfunction.

This situation can leave the heart attack survivor with a sense of anxiety and a sense of impending doom.

"Was that a twinge in my chest?" ......Indigestion.

"My left arm feels like it is tingling!"......I slept on it.

"I feel my heat beating faster for no reason!".....I have just eaten a big meal.

Now if this doesn't make you anxious and depressed nothing will.

And all this extra anxiety is just contributing to the risk.

The reality is, along with stress management strategies such as meditation, gratitude, yoga, saunas, etc we can start to adopt a practice of eradicating problematic lifestyle factors every day, and replacing them with positive ones as much as we can.

If you have a stoic, dedicated, single-minded personality then living what might seem an essentially abstentious life may come easier to you, but for most it is more a case of working towards progress more slowly, and if you aren't used to this it can be difficult and dis-heartening.

The best strategy I can think of is to take this approach:

1. Be kind to yourself.

2. Create habits that make adhering to stress management activities easier

3. Break activities down into small steps and work towards improvement every day

4. If one day you can't achieve what you hoped for then just aim a little lower and try again

5. Don't be tough on yourself! Just try to improve a little every day.

The compound effect of this strategy will leave you feeling less stressed about the end goals you set for your new lifestyle.

You will feel less worried about the possibility of another heart event, and will feel generally happier and more in control of the progress you are making.

Avoiding the worry and stress post heart-attack is as much part of the recovery as anything else you can do, so try not to fall into a downward spiral of negative thoughts, or set yourself up to fail with big lifestyle changes.

The diagram below has helped me to simplify how to approach creating small daily, positive changes, that may have large positive health effects.

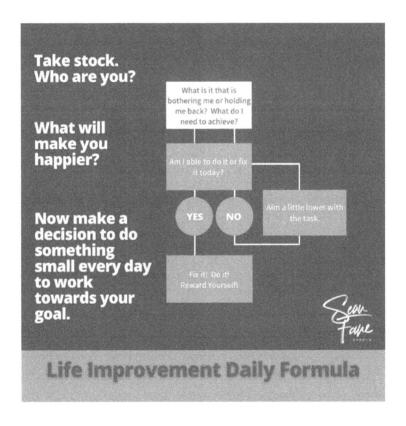

KNOW WHAT YOU ARE FIGHTING!

There are lots of different terms for heart disease.

As you may have gathered from reading through this book to this point, heart disease is a "catch-all" term for a variety of illnesses, mostly chronic, which develop over time and result in an "end-point" which might be labelled as a stroke or heart attack for simplicity.

You may also have gathered that there are myriad elements to the accumulation of challenges which will result in one of these heart disease end-points.

One person may suffer a myocardial infarction caused by the long-term effects of smoking and a poor diet.

Another may suffer the same fate through a genetic factor which increases their risk of blood clots and have a stressful job, which exacerbates the problem by increasing their blood pressure.

Each of us is different, and the factors that lead to us suffering (or not) at various points in our lives differ from person to person.

This is not much different to thinking about lung cancer and cigarette smoking.

Not everybody that smokes suffers from lung cancer. Some may smoke very little but contract lung cancer, others will smoke all of their lives and not contract lung cancer.

Each of us has different tolerances to the abuse that our bodies suffer, and a different genetic make-up which determines the extent to which our bodies respond to the foods, toxins and hormonal imbalances that we are exposed to.

Whilst there are some general lifestyle rules, which in combination can massively reduce future heart disease risk, by the time you have had a heart attack you should probably focus, quite specifically, on strengthening any particular weaknesses that you are more likely to encounter again.

This is the best strategy to buy yourself the time you need for a more thorough overall approach to new lifestyle implementations which will support a long and healthy life.

For example, there may be less benefit in quitting your stressful job if your individual susceptibility relates more closely with a high-glycemic diet which is taking you to the brink of type 2 diabetes. Clearly you would receive more immediate benefit from a dietary intervention.

That doesn't mean that reducing your stress isn't a good goal, but it might not be the first thing you would change.

In a previous chapter I have highlighted some tests which predict heart disease risk.

If it is not extremely clear to you what has caused your heart disease, then I would strongly suggest that you go through as much testing as possible until you find out what your weaknesses are, and then you can follow the right specific protocols to fix *your* underlying issues.

Accepting a statement like *"you are genetically susceptible"* or *"it runs in your family"* or *"it's likely to be a result of your weight"* or *"you have quite high cholesterol"* should **NEVER** be acceptable to you!

It is impossible to treat an *unspecified* problem effectively.

Get tested and know what you are fighting!

Summary

"If we don't change direction soon, we'll end up where we're going!"

— *Irwin Corey*

There is a great chapter in the Jordan B. Peterson book *12 Rules For Life* entitled **"Pursue What Is Meaningful (Not What Is Expedient)."**

Petersons explanation on the philosophy of instant gratification, and our ability to delay it, is extremely interesting.

It helps to understand why it can be so hard to do what we know we need to do to thrive and enjoy our lives to their fullest potential.

In the chapter he explains that many of us delay gratification every day without noticing it, for example when we go to work. The "employed" have essentially made a bargain with their employer….to sacrifice their time now, in order to improve their future earnings.

How does this relate to heart-disease?

Well, there is a definite link between chronic disease and lifestyle.

We seem to be "wedded" to lifestyles chosen for us by other people or by society, social customs, companies, convenience and laziness.

Often we do what is easy, or accepted, even though we know there are better choices for our long-term health.

It is **normal** to eat bread because we see others in our society do it, but in another time or in another part of the world, maybe it would not seem so normal. Certainly, Inuits in Alaska haven't historically thought it normal to eat bread.

It is **easy** to cook pasta, but would it be better to spend a little time planning a healthier choice for dinner and taking more time?

Summary

Eating sandwiches is _accepted_ by society as a norm, because nobody questions your food decisions when you have sandwiches for lunch. But is it better to eat something that supports our health, but which might raise a few eyebrows?

We grab a bar of chocolate at the till of the supermarket, because they have intentionally made easy and obvious and because we have trained our taste-buds to like sweet things. We are that easily influenced! (Anyone that has ever gone through the process of reducing sugar in tea, knows that once you adapt your tastebuds, having sugar afterwards tastes awful). We can train our tastebuds to like or dislike anything.

We can train our tastebuds to like or dislike anything.

So we know that societal norms choose our lifestyles for us….unless we decide to take a conscious decision to take control of our lifestyles ourselves.

And we can change our lifestyles if we want to, but it takes a strong goal.

Being a vegan is a great example of this.

Vegans make a decision not to eat animal products, and because it is linked to their ethics, moral standards and who they perceive themselves to "be" (which means they base their self-worth on it) they are generally very good at sticking to their lifestyle changes.

Having a strong goal, based on self-worth, and having it reflect who you are, is very powerful.

I am not advocating being a vegan, but the act of identifying as somebody that has a strong goal, you may develop a vegan-like ability to keep on track with your lifestyle choices.

Maybe making it associated with your sense of "self" will make it easier to reach that goal.

"I *am* committed to my health, so I ***don't*** eat high glycemic foods!" is a much more powerful statement of who you are than "I can't eat chocolate because I am on a diet!", which sounds like you are oppressed and depriving yourself of something.

This relates to heart health, because now you need to decide what you are prepared to do about your lifestyle to mitigate your future heart disease risk.

Throughout this book I have shared what causes heart disease, and how you can make changes to your lifestyle to either prevent heart disease from establishing itself, or reverse some of the symptoms if it has already affected you.

What should be crystal clear to you now, is that if you have a "normal" modern lifestyle, doing nothing....changing nothing.....you are essentially relying on chance.

You are gambling that you will be lucky enough to reach a significant age before the incremental effects of your/our lifestyle's trajectory towards chronic illnesses, such as cancer, Alzheimer's, dementia, type 2 diabetes, stroke and heart attack catch-up with you.

Have you won the genetic lottery?

Will you get away with it?

Like the smoker that believes he will never get lung cancer....there is a chance that you might.

Maybe your body can cope with lifestyle damage long enough.

We can choose to maintain the status quo. We can live for todays pleasure, or normality, or ease and tell ourselves that tomorrow's pain may not come.

Maybe your genetics give you enough head-start that disease won't catch you, and you will live to a fantastic age with no health repercussions. Some people do.

Summary

Maybe like me, you have a genetic weakness that means even relatively small lifestyle indiscretions will be punished.

Or maybe, like the majority of the population, you will succumb to these diseases in the Autumn of your years, and either suffer tragically with chronic poor health, or have an "event" that takes you suddenly from your loved-ones.

One thing is for sure, we have the power to control much of the outcome.

It is clear from human behaviour that if we don't see the *pain* in our *immediate future* with *absolute certainty* then we consistently fail to take action.

Do you see the potential for pain, sickness and death for you?

- If you feel healthy, probably not.

- If you are under 40, probably not.

- If you aren't overweight, probably not.

If you don't then you may feel unwilling to take action now for an outcome you don't anticipate happening.

But look at your 9 closest, healthy friends, and know that 7 of you will die from a chronic illness that will be lifestyle related.

Cancer, heart disease, stroke, diabetes, Alzheimer's disease or dementia.

We already know that in the "Western" world 1 in 2 adults is diabetic or pre-diabetic.

1 person every 36 seconds dies from heart disease in America. 655,000 people a year.

An estimated 17.9 million people died from CVD in 2016, representing 31% of all global deaths…almost all of those from heart-attacks and stroke.

Since 1996 the number of people diagnosed with diabetes in the UK has increased from 1.4million to 2.6 million, and many, many more remain un-diagnosed or pre-diabetic.

These are shocking statistics for a "civilised" world, and they are getting worse!

Not only that, but the quality of our lives diminishes gradually at first and then accelerates towards the end of our lives, when we allow chronic disease to become an acceptable part of the ageing process.

Instead of maintaining good health to actually enjoy our lives, many of us spend our last 10, 20 or even 30 years suffering in pain, sick and medicated as a consequence of the chronic illnesses our lifestyles create.

We prematurely become unable to participate in the activities that we love, like snowboarding, playing tennis or golf….or even walking for any distance, as the consequences of chronic modern diseases, and the medications we take to treat them, rob us of our strength and vitality and our general health declines.

Summary

THE LIFE IN YOUR YEARS
QUALITY OF LIFE OVER YOUR LIFESPAN

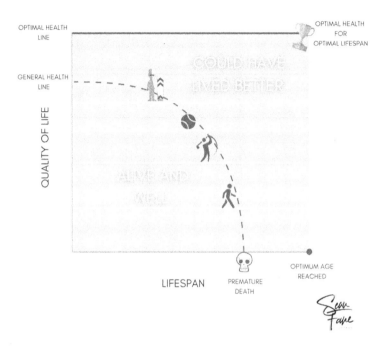

Could we live longer lives with more quality of life, fit and active, with no fear of diabetes, Alzheimer's, CVD and dementia?

Surely it is better to sacrifice some of the pleasure we may derive from sugar, vegetable oil, cigarettes, bread, rice, pasta, crisps and lounging in-front of the sofa, to live a longer life with robust health?

Is that even a sacrifice? Or is it just "re-wiring" ourselves so that our pleasures are no longer killing us slowly, but are instead improving our vitality.

Is it not worth the delayed gratification of making a few swaps, like replacing "poisons" such as sugar, wheat and processed food with grass-fed beef, eggs, milk, butter, cream and the great outdoors for a life, lived to a ripe-old age, full of energy?

We can't mitigate against every negative health outcome with lifestyle, but we can start to live a life that makes it much less likely that we will be taken early or suffer for decades.

What would it take for you to make lifestyle changes now, that come to feel normal, natural and easy over time, and prevent the need for assisted living, drug dependence and pain later?

If we start to live a life that becomes the new "normal", then maybe generations to come will avoid the mistakes that the last few generations have made.

Maybe our children, and our children's children will benefit from the changes we make, and have longer, healthier happier lives themselves.

Who wouldn't want that?

Thank you for reading Use Your Head, Heal Your Heart.

I hope it has helped to inform you, and unravel some of the complexity of heart disease, and I hope it helps you steer a path to great health.

WHAT ARE THE WARNING SIGNS THAT YOU MAY BE HAVING A HEART ATTACK?

These warning signs do not necessarily mean that you are having a heart attack, but if you start to experience one or more of these symptoms, and you don't have another logical explanation, make sure you get tested for risk.

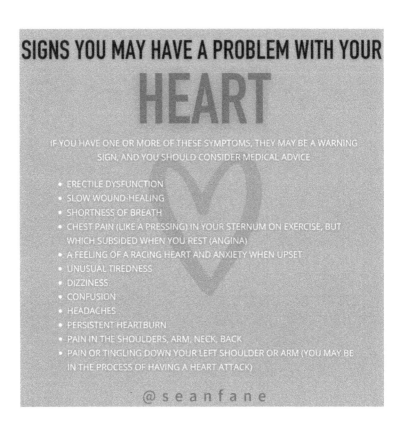

This little tip could be a life-saver…if you think you are having a heart attack, then chew on an aspirin and call 999 immediately.

Get the ambulance to hospital, DON'T DRIVE!

NB. I made the mistake of being driven to hospital by my partner Julie, and upon explaining that I had had a heart attack, was made to sit in a queue in the reception area for two hours while people with cuts and bruises were triaged before me, as they arrived earlier!

Had I called the ambulance I would have received immediate treatment en-route and would have been taken straight to the cardiac ward.

Always call an ambulance!

SUPPLEMENTS

I have noted a few key supplements that can really aid recovery after a heart attack, or if you think you have risk factors that you would like to manage better.

This is not an exhaustive list, but will provide you with a good idea as to which supplements might aid you on your personal journey of great health and recovery.

- *Vitamin B5* (Pantothenic acid) - Has a positive impact on triglycerides and LDL cholesterol pattern[44]. It also increases HDL. *It can be found in beef, chicken, organ meats, mushrooms and avocado so if you eat sufficient quantities of these foods then I would not supplement. If your dietary intake is insufficient and you have a high blood triglyceride measurement (and these two things might tell you that you need to change your diet) then supplementation can help to address blood lipids.*

- *Citrus Bergamot* - It can lower blood sugar, lower triglycerides, raise HDL and reduce LP(a) in some people. It can help with those with pre-diabetes[45]. *I have seen rec-*

---

44 https://www.hsph.harvard.edu/nutritionsource/pantothenic-acid-vitamin-b5/

45 https://www.ncbi.nlm.nih.gov/pmc/articles/PMC6497409/

ommended 650mg twice per day if you have significant insulin resistance or are diagnosed as pre-diabetic.

- *Vitamin C* - All animals, with only a few exceptions, produce large quantities of vitamin C in their bodies (2- 20 grams /day) to support optimum collagen production necessary for maintaining healthy and elastic blood vessels. High levels of endogenous vitamin C production protects animals arteries from damage and development of atherosclerotic deposits. This is why animals do not die of heart attacks, even if some of them, such as bears, have very high blood cholesterol levels (600 mg/dl). In contrast, humans lost our ability to produce vitamin C and our daily dietary intake is often insufficient for optimum vascular health. **The RDA for vitamin C is 60-80 mg/day, which is ridiculously LOW!!** *I take at least 2,000 to 4,000 mg per day, and would suggest more might be appropriate for those with elevated genetic LP(a). The liposomal vitamin C from Altrient[46] is very highly absorbed, and is exceptional quality.*

- *Coco Flavanols* - Found in dark chocolate, they lower blood pressure and stimulate nitric oxide production. *I regularly consume low, or zero, sugar very dark chocolate and have acquired a taste for it. It can be grated onto yoghurt or added to ketogenic cheesecake recipes.*

---

[46]   www.altrient.com

Supplements

- ***Co-Enzyme Q10*** - It is made in every cell in the body. It creates energy from food. The human body can't work without it. The heart is one of the organs where the most Co-Enzyme Q10 is concentrated (the other is the liver). We create less as we age, but it is as important to the heart as calcium is to bones. The only foods you can eat that contain significant amounts are organ meats such as heart and liver. **Statins deplete Co-Enzyme Q10 levels, and this is one of the reasons people can suffer with weakness and muscle pain when taking statins.** The mevalonate pathway (that produces cholesterol) also produces Co-Enzyme Q10. When you block this pathway (this is what statins actually do) you reduce the body's ability to produce cholesterol and also Co-Enzyme Q10. For this reason, **anyone on statins MUST supplement with Co-Enzyme Q10**. It is so important it has been approved in Japan on prescription for congestive heart failure. It is also able to reduce blood pressure. It is a powerful anti-oxidant, inhibiting oxidative damage to LDL cholesterol. It has a symbiotic relationship with vitamin E. In rats Vitamin E has been proven to increase blood levels of Co-Enzyme Q10. In baboons given C0-Enzyme Q10, the anti-inflammatory effects of vitamin E were increased. In one study Co-Enzyme Q10 plus vitamin E lowered HS-CRP. Lastly…it reduces LP(a) which is one of the most significant factors in genetic heart disease risk. *I take 100 to 300mg per day of the* ubiquinol *version.*

- ***Creatine Monohydrate*** - Creatine is a substance that is found naturally in muscle cells. It helps your muscles produce energy. It is abundant in red meat, and can also be created in our body from a combination of amino acids. It improves cell signalling, raises metabolic hormones, increases cell hydration, prevents protein breakdown and lowers levels of myostatin (a protein that can inhibit muscle growth). *This is all good news for your heart. I add creatine and L-carnitine into a whey protein shake for a daily boost for muscle strength (your heart is a muscle too!).*

- *Vitamin D* - Vitamin D reverses insulin resistance and is anti-inflammatory. It improves bone health and the immune system, and is vital for so many gene expressions that it would take another book to list them! Crucial for good health! *I take 2,000 to 3,000 IU's per day as a minimum (30,000 IU's per day for a few days if I become ill or am deficient and need to kick-start raising my circulating blood levels).*

- *D-Ribose* - D-Ribose improves the hearts ability to tolerate low blood flow[47], so is ideal for those that have already suffered heart disease. It also helps with energy production in muscle and plays an enormous part in restoring diastolic function. *I take 5 to 60g per day in a protein shake.*

- *Vitamin E* - Vitamin E is a powerful anti-oxidant, usually formed from mixed tocopherols and tocotrienols. Vitamin E is over-hyped and under-delivers in my opinion, so unless you are deficient, I would not suggest you supplement. You get plenty of vitamin E when your diet is healthy. Foods such as eggs, nuts, bell-peppers, spinach and greens contain vitamin E.

---

[47] https://www.thelancet.com/journals/lancet/article/PII0140-6736(92)91709-H/fulltext

Supplements

- *Garlic* - Lowers lipids, is anti-thrombotic and reduces blood coagulation. *I would suggest 600 to 1,200mg per day as a supplement if you have clotting related challenges.*

- *Vitamin K2* - An essential nutrient. Many people, including doctors, confuse K2 with K1 (a vitamin involved in clotting). Few people are deficient in K1 as it is easily obtained from the diet and gets recycled in the body. K2, however, is a lot harder to obtain. It is the "traffic-policeman" for calcium, directing it *out* of soft tissue (like arteries), and *in* to bones and teeth, where it should be. Additionally, it 'activates' many proteins in the body, and dietary intake of K2 has been linked with reduced cancer incidence, increased insulin sensitivity, better brain health, and more. If you want to learn more about how vitamin K2 helps to reverse atherosclerosis (and it is fascinating, but quite technical) then visit the website of Patrick Theut at www.k-vitamins.com. The world's highest dietary source of K2 is found in something called natto. *If you have known arterial calcification I suggest taking 'Koncentrated K' from the website noted.*

- *L-Carnitine* - Supplementation after a heart attack, increases survival rate and makes it less likely that you will suffer a subsequent heart attack. Works with Co-Enzyme Q10 to facilitate the production of ATP. *I suggest taking 1,500 to 2,500mg per day if you have already experienced a heart attack.*

- *Lumbrokinase* - In 1991, Dr. Mihara, and other scientists in Japan, successfully extracted and characterized a group of fibrinolytic enzymes from earthworms (yes really) called *Lumbricus Rubellus*. These enzymes are capable of degrading both plasminogen-rich and plasminogen-free fibrin. So they break-down fibrinogen, which is a substance that causes blood clots. *If you have high levels of fibrinogen, and are prone to blood clots, this is a supplement worth consideration (even if it sounds unpalatable).*

- *Magnesium* - Relaxes artery walls, reduces blood pressure. It reverses endothelial dysfunction by interacting with calcium. *I take 400mg per day.*

- *Nattokinase* - This is an enzyme that is extracted from a popular Japanese food called natto. Natto is boiled soybeans that have been fermented with a type of bacteria. Nattokinase lowers blood-pressure, has anti-artherosclerotic effects and lowers blood lipids. It has also shown potential for degrading Alzheimer's-related plaques. This astonishing supplement was described in this 2018 scholarly article[48] in glowing terms; *"Compared with traditional antithrombotic and antihypertensive drugs, nattokinase is characterised by high safety, low cost, simple production process, oral availability, and long in vivo half-life". "As such, it is expected to become a new-generation drug for thrombotic disorders or CVD".*

- *Niacin (B3)* - Lowers triglycerides and LDL pattern B cholesterol. **Reduces LP(a) and raises HDL.** *I take 1,000 mg per day. Don't use timed-release.*

---

[48]   https://www.ncbi.nlm.nih.gov/pmc/articles/PMC6043915/

Supplements

- *Olive Leaf Complex* - Lowers blood pressure. *1,000mg per day has been shown to reduce systolic figures by 11 points over an 8-week period[49].*

- *Omega 3* - It is highly anti-inflammatory, and is found mainly in oily fish. Heart super-supplement Omega 3 lowers blood-pressure, reduces triglycerides and slows plaque development in arteries. We have so much Omega 6 oil from appalling "vegetable" oils, that our requirement for Omega 3 (they balance each other out) is much increased. *I take 1000 mg per day.*

- *Potassium* - Found in seeds like flax as well as dark chocolate, avocados, nuts and fatty fish. Potassium balances sodium, and should be maintained through diet.

- *Probiotic* - Probiotics can help to reduce blood pressure and have been shown to improve blood sugar levels. They re-populate good bacteria, and support immune function as well as good mental health. Taking the right probiotic is important. Opt for quality, not quantity. *Choose Rhamnosus, Bifidum (helps digest dairy), Longum, Acidophilus (helps nutrient absorption) and Fermentum.*

- *Resveratrol* - Protects against blood clots, reduces blood pressure. Powerful anti-oxidant. *I take 200mg per day.*

49
https://www.sciencedirect.com/science/article/abs/pii/S09447113
10002709

- *Zinc* - Studies have shown links between zinc levels and cardiac health [50]. Concentrations of glutathione and vitamin E in the heart muscle decline alongside the bodies´ zinc status. These are powerful antioxidants, so in addition to essential metabolic functions, the level of zinc in the body also affects the heart muscle's ability to combat oxidative stress. Great sources of zinc are red meat, shellfish, peanuts, cashews, almonds, chickpeas, dairy, lentils and eggs.

---

[50] https://www.sciencedaily.com/releases/2017/04/170418094238.htm

GLOSSARY

1. **AF** - Atrial fibrillation. When you have atrial fibrillation, you might notice a skipped heartbeat, and then feel a thud or thump, followed by your heart racing for an extended amount of time. You might feel heart palpitations or a fluttering/jumping of your heart. Experiencing sweating or chest pain is also common. It is possible to have an atrial fibrillation episode that resolves on its own, but it may be a persistent condition that requires treatment. Stress, high blood pressure and a number of other factors can cause AF. If you feel yourself suffering from these symptoms, try to relax, drink plenty of water and call for medical assistance. AF increases risk of stroke or heart failure.

2. **Angina** - Often referred to as stable angina. Pain or tightness in the chest. Brought on most often when angry, anxious, during physical exertion. This lasts for a few minutes up to a few hours, and is caused by a blockage which prevents the heart from receiving enough oxygen. Seek medical assistance if you experience angina!

3. **Unstable Angina** - The same symptoms as Angina, but appearing with no obvious triggers in the form of stress or physical exertion. Very dangerous and the precursor to a heart-attack. _Time to get to hospital!!_

4. **Angioplasty** - where a tube is threaded into an artery, and then inflated, to widen the vessel and increase blood flow.

5. **Antioxidants** - Oxidative stress has been linked to cancer, atherosclerosis, and vision loss. An intake of antioxidants is believed to reduce these risks. Antioxidants include things like vitamin A, vitamin C, vitamin E, beta-carotene, lycopene, lutein, selenium, manganese, zeaxanthin and resveratrol.

6. **ApoA1** - Apolipoprotein A1 is the primary protein component of high-density lipoprotein (HDL).

7. **ApoB** - Apolipoprotein B is the primary protein of VLDL, Lp(a) and low-density lipoprotein (LDL).

8. **APOe4** - is a protein involved in the metabolism of fats in the body of mammals.

9. **Atherosclerosis** - refers to the build-up of substances in your artery walls (plaque), which can restrict blood flow. The plaque can burst, triggering a blood clot. Although atherosclerosis is often considered a heart problem, it can affect arteries anywhere in your body.

10. **CAD** - Coronary Artery Disease. Angina, heart attacks and stroke often come under this description.

11. **CHD** - Coronary Heart Disease (see CAD).

12. Cardiac Arrest - A sudden loss of blood flow resulting from the failure of the heart to pump effectively. Like an electrical impulse malfunctioning. Signs include loss of consciousness and abnormal or absent breathing.

13. Chronic Inflammation - When the body is subjected to continual repeated harmful stimuli, the usually helpful, temporary healing process of inflammation becomes so persistent that it damages the otherwise healthy areas that are targeted.

14. CPR - Cardio Pulmonary Resuscitation. A medical procedure involving repeated cycles of compression of the chest, and artificial respiration, performed to maintain blood circulation and oxygenation in a person who has suffered cardiac arrest.

15. **CVD** - Cardio Vascular Disease is a general term for conditions affecting the heart or blood vessels. It's usually associated with a "thickening" of the inside the artery walls (atherosclerosis) and an increased risk of blood clots.

Glossary

16. **DAPT** - Dual Anti-Platelet Therapy is a term that refers to the practice of being prescribed both a blood thinner (such as aspirin) and anti-coagulant (much as Clopidogrel, Plavix) concurrently. This reduces the risks of clotting to a greater degree than either treatment alone.

17. **DES** - Drug Eluding Stents. These have built in anti-coagulant medications and enable the reduction or early cessation of prescribed anticoagulants. They reduce the risk or re-narrowing of the stent.

18. **Diastolic** - The second number in a blood pressure reading. The pressure when the heart relaxes and blood flows in.

19. **Endothelium** - Also known as the endothelial wall, is a layer of cells (only one cell thick generally) which are tiled to line the walls of arteries and veins and act as a first line of defence for the wall integrity.

20. **Familial Hypercholesterolemia** - A defect (mutation) in a gene changes how the body processes cholesterol. This mutation prevents the body from removing LDL cholesterol from the blood. This results in very high levels of cholesterol. In a chronic inflammatory environment having cholesterol levels this high is potentially dangerous.

21. **Fat** - Fat is a term used to describe a class of macro nutrients used in metabolism called triglycerides.

22. **Free Radicals** - Oxygen free radicals are created when an oxygen molecule splits into a single atom of unpaired electrons. They prefer to be in pairs, and cause damage to cells, protein and DNA when they bounce around looking for another electron to pair with. Anti-oxidants soak them-up.

23. **HDL** - High Density Lipoprotein. Referred to, by many, as "good cholesterol".

24. **HDL 2** - Large and protective molecules with anti-inflammatory properties.. Higher HDL 2 than 3 is better for health.

25. **HDL 3** - Small and dense molecules and may be inflammatory. A higher HDL 2 to HDL 3 ratio is required for good health.

26. **Inflammation** - The response of your body to harmful stimuli. Damaged cells, pathogens and other irritants stimulate a defence from your body which involves immune cells, blood vessels and other molecular aids.

27. **Insulin Resistance** - The term describing a cells lack of response to insulin. When this happens, our body produces more insulin to generate a response, which is harmful, creates a vicious-cycle of hormonal imbalance and can ultimately lead to many chronic health conditions including type 2 diabetes and heart disease.

28. **LAD** - Left Anterior Descending. Known as "The Widow-Maker" as it is the most important artery serving the left ventricle of the heart with blood, and if it is blocked there is little time to perform an intervention.

29. **LDL** - Low Density Lipoprotein. Referred to, by many, as "bad cholesterol".

30. **LDL Pattern A** - A configuration where more of the smaller, atherogenic particles make-up the bulk of a person's LDL total.

31. **LDL Pattern B** - A configuration where more of the larger, benign particles make-up the bulk of a person's LDL total.

32. **LP(a)** - Lipoprotein A (also known as LP "little" a or "sticky cholesterol") is a particle in the blood that is part of the LDL family, and is made by the liver. It is basically LDL with apolipoprotein A attached. The amount one makes is determined by genetics. 20-30% of people have inherited high levels

of LP(a) production, and it can dramatically increase the likelihood of a heart attack. LP(a) fights collagen breakdown, but in the process creates un-dissolvable clots, where blood vessel walls are damaged (sometimes a consequence of a vitamin C deficiency). *Niacin and vitamin B3 have been shown to lower LP(a). Vitamin C supplementation may prevent collagen breakdown, and subsequent LP(a) activation in clotting.*

33. *Metabolic Syndrome* - This is a term used to describe the collective effect of insulin resistance and the mechanisms that cause your body to fail to regulate your hormones. (See Insulin Resistance).

34. *MINOCA* - Myocardial Infarction with Non-Obstructed Coronary Arteries. A strange event where a heart attack with all the symptoms is experienced but where no blockage can be found.

35. *Mono-Unsaturated Fat* - Fatty acids with one double bond.

36. *Myocardial Infarction* - Another way of saying a heart attack! Where the myocardial ischemia lasts too long or is severe and causes a plaque rupture it is referred to as infarction. *Symptoms include chest pain, tingling or discomfort in shoulder, back, neck or jaw.*

37. *Myocardial Ischemia* - Simply the blood flow decreasing dramatically, or stopping completely to a part of the heart.

38. *N-STEMI* - Non-ST-Segment Elevation Myocardial Infarction. An NSTEMI can be less serious than a STEMI because the supply of blood to the heart may be only partially, rather than completely, blocked. As a result, a smaller section of the heart may be damaged. However, an N-STEMI is still regarded as a serious medical emergency.

39. *Omega 3* - There are three main types of Omega 3 that we consume. ALA, EPA and DHA. Many studies have assessed

the effects of omega-3s—primarily EPA and DHA—on cardiovascular disease and risk factors such as high blood pressure and elevated plasma lipids. This was originally noted after anecdotally discovering low rates of coronary events among Greenland Inuit and other fish-eating populations. Results from observational studies have been consistent with these findings, with several systematic reviews and meta-analyses showing that higher consumption of fish and higher dietary or plasma levels of omega-3s are associated with a lower risk of heart failure, coronary disease, and fatal coronary heart disease. ALA, found in seeds and plants can be converted into EPA and then to DHA, by your liver, but the conversion is inefficient and only 5% to 15% is actually generated through this process. For these reasons, consuming EPA and DHA directly from foods or dietary supplements is the only practical way to increase levels of Omega 3 fatty acids in your body.

40. *Omega 6* - A family of polyunsaturated fatty acids that have in common a final carbon-carbon double bond in the n-6 position. Chronic excessive production of omega-6 is correlated with arthritis, inflammation, and cancer.

41. *Oxidation* - The process of damage caused by free radical activity.

42. *Oxidative stress* - The damage caused by free radical activity.

43. *PCI* - Percutaneous Coronary Intervention. This is another way of referring to one of the two treatments for artery blockage. One is the insertion of a "stent" the other is the inflation of a balloon to clear a blockage. The process is similar for both and is called a PCI.

44. *Poly-Unsaturated Fat* - Fatty acids with two or more double bonds.

45. **_PE_** - pulmonary embolism is a term to describe a clot that travels through the blood system and gets stuck in the lungs.

46. **_Saturated Fat_** - Much demonised fatty acids with mainly single bonds. They tend to be solid at room temperature. Great for cooking as they are stable when heated. **_Found in meats, lard, full-fat dairy products (butter, cream) coconuts, coconut oil, palm oil, dark chocolate. Fill Your Boots!_**

47. **_"Silent" MI_** - A heart attack with no symptoms and where the sufferer doesn't even notice they have had a heart attack. More common in women, the elderly and those with diabetes.

48. **_STEMI_** - ST-Segment Elevation Myocardial Infarction. Most serious form of heart attack where the blockage is complete to a major artery. Extensive heart damage is likely.

49. **_Stent_** - A small mesh tube that is inserted into an artery and pushed open, at the site of a narrowing, with a small balloon during an angioplasty. It stays in the artery keeping it open.

50. **_Stroke_** - Ischaemic stroke is where atherosclerotic plaque generates a blood clot in the carotid artery that breaks off and travels to the brain where it gets stuck and creates a cerebral infarction. Haemorrhaging strokes are where a blood vessel bursts in the brain, and are often caused by high blood pressure.

51. **_Systolic_** - The first number on a blood pressure reading, when the heart squeezes and pumps out blood.

52. **_Takotsubo Syndrome_** - Almost all the signs of a heart attack but where there is no blood clot and no infarction, yet people may still die from it. It is sometimes referred to as "dying of a broken heart" as it can brought-on by sudden emotional stress.

53. **_tPA_** - tissues plasminogen activator is a term for treatment of an infarction by breaking down blood clots.

54. ***Trans Fat*** - These fats are created when vegetable oils are chemically altered to remain solid at room temperature. They are added to processed foods to lengthen shelf-life and to add texture. ***"High trans fat consumption remains a significant risk factor for CHD".***[51]

55. ***Vegetable Oil*** - A generic term for oils, high in omega 6 fatty acids, derived from a variety of seeds and fruits…but almost never vegetables.

56. ***VF*** - Ventricular Fibrillation is the most common type of "electrical" malfunction, where the heart loses its beating rhythm and causes a cardiac arrest.

---

[51]   https://pubmed.ncbi.nlm.nih.gov/17389261/

REFERENCES & FURTHER READING

I would like to acknowledge all of the amazing authors and educators that have influenced my journey of discovery, the eradication of propaganda and development of knowledge that has led to me writing this book.

For those that want to delve deeper, learn the science (not just the concepts) and understand more of the history of chronic disease, I highly recommend the following books, podcasts, articles, experts and reference sources.

Books Referenced:

The Greater Cholesterol Myth - Johnny Bowden PhD CNS , Steven Sinatra MD FACC

A Statin Nation - Dr Malcolm Kendrick

The Great Cholesterol Con - Dr Malcolm Kendrick

Doctoring Data - Dr Malcolm Kendrick

The Big Fat Surprise - Nina Tiecholz

The Case Against Sugar - Gary Taubes

Pure, White & Deadly - John Yudkin

The Dark Side of Statins - The Wonder Of Cholesterol - Duane Graveline MD, MPH

Why We Get Sick - Benjamin Bikman PhD

Why Animals Don't Get Heart Attacks - But People Do! - Dr Matthius Rath MD

Statins Toxic Side Effects - Evidence From 500 Scientific Papers - David Evans

Low Cholesterol Leads To An Early Death - Evidence From 101 Scientific Papers - David Evans

Cholesterol And Saturated Fat Prevent Heart Disease - Evidence From 101 Scientific Papers - David Evans

The Fat Emperor Podcast - Ivor Cummins

Unconventional Medicine - Chris Kresser

Put Your Heart In Your Mouth - Natasha Campbell-McBride

The Longevity Roadmap (Docu-Series) - Mark Hyman

The Diabetes Code - Jason Fung

The Cholesterol Hypothesis - Dr Tim Noakes

Glow 15 - Naomi Whittle

The Optimal Dose - Dr Judson Somerville

Atomic Habits - James Clear

12 Rules For Life - Jordan Peterson

Social Media Accounts To Follow:

Instagram @seanfane – (Me) Resources to help you manage your heart health

Instagram @rubiofuerte - Nutritional advice made simple

Instagram @maxlugavere - Science-based health and dietary advice

Instagram @healthcoachkait - Ketogenic diet advice and nutritional information made simple

Instagram @drstephenhussey - Functional medicine and heart health author

Instagram @meowmeix - Food facts and recipes for optimal health

Facebook Page - Use Your Head, Heal Your Heart

Facebook Page - Statins - The Silent Killer

Facebook Page - SugarByHalf

Facebook Page - Sugar Me Intolerant and Carb Me Sick "Low Carb Sensibility"

Facebook Page - Lower Insulin

CPSIA information can be obtained
at www.ICGtesting.com
Printed in the USA
BVHW080013150521
607367BV00001B/125